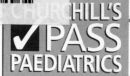

✓ **PASS**
PAEDIATRICS
CHURCHILL'S

WS18.2
WIN

Imaging
Pic
for
M

For Michael and Sophie

Commissioning Editor: Ellen Green
Project Manager: Fiona Young
Design direction: Erik Bigland/Judith Wright

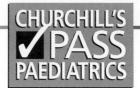

Imaging Picture Tests for the MRCPCH

A. P. Winrow
BSc(Hons) MB BS MRCP(UK) FRCPCH
Consultant Paediatrician, Kingston Hospital,
Kingston upon Thames, Surrey

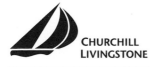

CHURCHILL
LIVINGSTONE

EDINBURGH LONDON NEW YORK PHILADELPHIA ST LOUIS SYDNEY TORONTO 2000

CHURCHILL LIVINGSTONE
An imprint of Harcourt Publishers Limited

© Harcourt Publishers Limited 2000

 is a registered trademark of Harcourt Publishers Limited

The right of Dr A P Winrow to be identified as author of this work has
been asserted by him in accordance with the Copyright, Designs and
Patents Act 1988

First published 2000

ISBN 0 443 06445 8

British Library Cataloguing in Publication Data
A catalogue record for this book is available from the British Library

Library of Congress Cataloging in Publication Data
A catalog record for this book is available from the Library of Congress

Note
Medical knowledge is constantly changing. As new information
becomes available, changes in treatment, procedures, equipment and
the use of drugs become necessary. The author and the publishers have,
as far as it is possible, taken care to ensure that the information given in
this text is accurate and up-to-date. However, readers are strongly
advised to confirm that the information, especially with regard to drug
usage, complies with the latest legislation and standards of practice.

The
publisher's
policy is to use
paper manufactured
from sustainable forests

Printed in China

Preface

It is customary to preface a postgraduate examination text with a statement that exams are a necessary evil. Unfortunately, this is no consolation for the beleaguered candidate who is trying to master a multitude of facts as well as combine theoretical knowledge with clinical experience in answering the examination question. It is hoped that this book will help with this problem.

The book contains radiological cases prepared in a manner seen in the MRCPCH Part 2 examination. Imaging studies are frequently encountered in all areas of the examination, not just the photographic material section. A wide range of disorders, radiological examinations and radiological features are considered in the book. It is envisaged that this will be a useful addition to the candidate's revision programme. Key facts relating to the case, including both clinical and radiological features as well as examination tips, are discussed alongside the relevant answers. This is not a text of paediatric radiology – nor, as a practising paediatrician, would I have the audacity to compile such a text. It is a book of paediatric images for trainee paediatricians facing the major examination of their careers. The cases cannot be exhaustive but they do cover a wide cross-section of potential MRCPCH topics. The discussion sections should act as a prompt to ensure that candidates refresh their knowledge of the disorders by reading more detailed articles.

The majority of the cases and questions have been tested on my junior colleagues in the past and I thank them for their comments. I hope that candidates find that the book is a helpful and stimulating way to gain further experience in the examination-orientated interpretation of imaging studies as well as an enjoyable test of their knowledge.

APW

Acknowledgements

I thank my colleagues, particularly Dr Richard Wilson and Dr Sinan Al-Jawad at Kingston Hospital, for their forbearance over the years when I have requested the opportunity to arrange copies of radiological investigations performed on their patients. The constructive comments of students and junior colleagues have always been enlightening.

I would also like to thank all at Harcourt Publishers for their support, advice and enthusiasm in enabling the completion of this project.

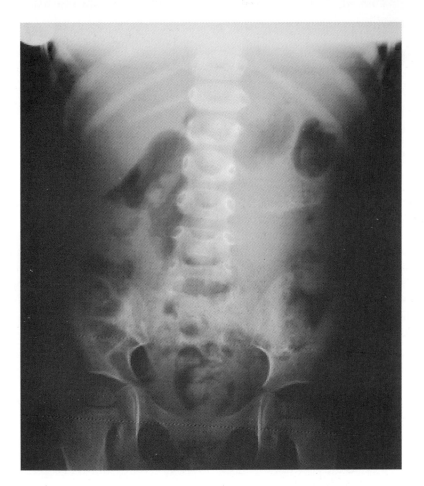

This 2-year-old girl was referred with abdominal discomfort and a 3-week history of refusal to weight-bear. An abdominal X-ray was performed.

a) What abnormality is demonstrated?
b) What is the most likely diagnosis?
c) List three additional investigations to aid diagnosis.

ANSWER 1

a) Speckled calcification in the left upper side of the abdomen which does not cross the midline.

b) Left abdominal neuroblastoma.

c) Further imaging of abdomen, either abdominal CT scan or abdominal ultrasound scan.
Urinary catecholamine assay.
Biopsy with cytogenetic analysis.
Methyliodobenzoguanidine (MIBG) isotope scan.
Bone marrow aspiration.

Comments

- A common examination scenario both as a clinical photograph and 'grey case' - always consider both neuroblastoma and acute leukaemia as differential diagnoses in a child with a limp or refusal to weight-bear alongside more obvious diagnoses such as trauma.
- Neuroblastoma remains the most common extracranial solid tumour in children, affecting about 1 in 7000 children below the age of 5 years
- Approximately 65% present in the abdomen, with a posterior mediastinal thoracic presentation in 20%.
- Other tumour effects may include compression of other structures, dissemination (including into bone) and constitutional effects. Survival correlates with stage and molecular characteristics. Remember the prognosis of infants with stage IV S is usually good.
- As a neural crest-derived tumour, it may arise along the paravertebral sympathetic chain.
- MIBG isotope is preferentially accumulated by neural crest-derived tissue, thereby aiding both diagnosis, disease monitoring and treatment.

Examination tips

- Be as specific as possible i.e. state left side.
- Think of an adrenal tumour if an intravenous urogram (IVU) picture is shown with evidence of compression of the kidney or dye – it may be a compression by an adrenal mass.
- Check whether the calcification is heterogeneous and whether it crosses the midline.
- Check for hepatomegaly on the X-ray.

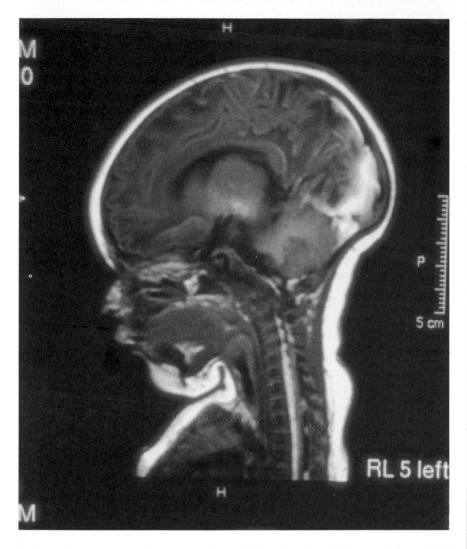

A 38-week gestation infant was admitted directly after delivery with marked respiratory distress. The infant suddenly deteriorated clinically. Apnoeic episodes occurred followed by generalised seizures. This MRI scan was obtained. The delivery had been prolonged and difficult with evidence of fetal distress on the cardiotocograph.

a) What is the most likely diagnosis?
b) In what other situations is this seen?
c) What is the likely causative mechanism?

ANSWER 2

a) Posterior fossa subdural haemorrhage.
b) Non-accidental injury.
   Road traffic accident trauma.
   Coagulopathy, e.g. haemorrhagic disease of the newborn.
c) This is caused by rapid stretching of bridging veins crossing the subdural space during delivery.

Comments
- Central nervous system (CNS) causes of respiratory distress are relatively uncommon.
- Apnoea may be due to CNS disease – the timing of this presentation indicates a recent onset of the problem; the history suggests a perinatal problem.
- Bridging veins are easy to rupture and can result in extensive bleeding.
- Cranial ultrasound is not the best modality for identifying subdural haemorrhage or problems confined to the posterior fossa.
- Subarachnoid haemorrhage may also occur spontaneously during delivery. The subsequent presentation is of an unexpectedly floppy infant.

Examination tips
- MRI scans may now be included in the examination – try to review as many as possible.
- This scan shows blood as a bright white high signal.
- Do not panic when faced with a MRI scan. Review it in a manner similar to that undertaken with a CT scan. In particular, compare sides if this is available.

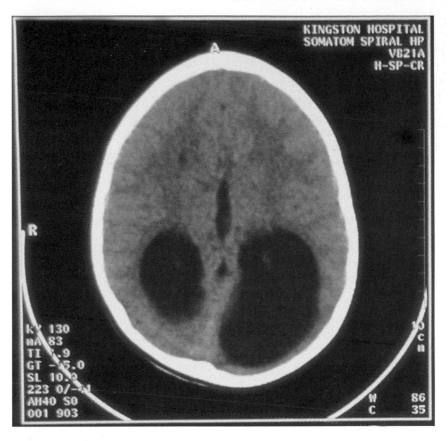

Emma, aged 7 years, was referred with episodes of pallor and non-specific headaches. A CT cranial scan was performed.

a) What is the most likely diagnosis?
b) List two other potential clinical associations which may coexist.

ANSWER 3

a) Dysgenesis of the corpus callosum.
b) Neurodevelopmental delay.
   Learning problems.
   Seizures of various types.

Comments

- Dysgenesis of the corpus callosum is a rare central nervous system structural anomaly. There is a spectrum of abnormality from partial (dysgenesis) to agenesis. The latter may be isolated or may be part of a wider disorder such as Aicardi syndrome.
- Large interhemispheric cysts are rare associations.
- The degree of neurological or neurodevelopmental deficit is difficult to predict and the prognosis in some individuals is very good.
- Seizures are frequently associated.

Examination tips

- CT cranial scans are often encountered in the examination.
- DO NOT PANIC – look logically, comparing both sides and not forgetting the interface between brain and skull.
- If in difficulty, try to describe what you can see, succinctly, accurately and logically.

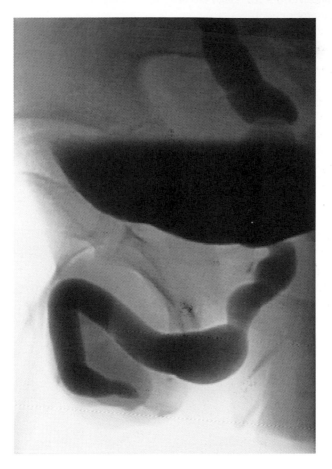

Richard, aged 14 years, was referred having suffered dysuria and haematuria. The illustrated investigation was performed.

a) What investigation has been performed?
b) List three radiological abnormalities.
c) What is the most likely abnormality?

ANSWER 4

a) Intravenous urogram (IVU) (screening image).
b) Hydroureter.
  Hypertrophied/dilated bladder.
  Dilated urethra.
  Distal meatal stenosis.
c) Obstructive uropathy secondary to meatal stenosis.

Comments

- The whole urinary system that is shown is dilated. This must be proximal to the obstruction. When the bladder appears dilated, both a posterior urethral valve problem and a neuropathic bladder must be considered in the differential diagnosis.
- The whole of the urethra is dilated except for the terminal meatus.
- The ureter is dilated due to back pressure, resulting in hydroureter and nephropathy – the latter is not demonstrated on this film. A renal ultrasound scan showed bilateral irregular scarring which was translated into poor function on a DMSA isotope scan. Treatment was a meatoplasty.

Examination tips

- Always orientate yourself – check where the radio-opaque dye is outlining.
- Look for clues to the anatomy if possible, e.g. bony structures.
- Many candidates have identified this as a barium enema – don't panic if you did as well!
- This is an IVU *not a micturating cystourethrogram* (MCUG), as the bladder is not fully filled as it would appear in a MCUG.
- Always look in the corners of the picture – this reveals the thin line of dye in the distal meatus.

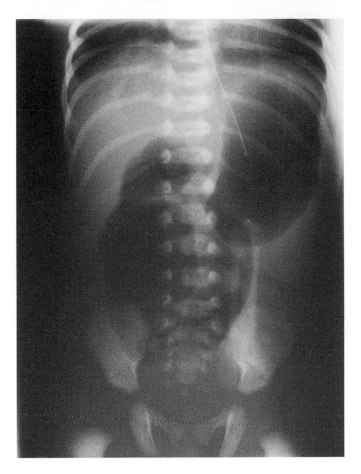

A neonate, aged 6 hours, is admitted to the neonatal intensive care with bile-stained vomiting. He was born at term after a normal delivery. No abnormal antenatal history was apparent from maternal notes.

a) Describe the abnormality demonstrated.
b) What is the probable diagnosis?

ANSWER 5

a) Multiple loops of distended gut – in this case three loops.
b) Jejunal atresia.

Comments

- Both in the examination and (usually) in practice, bile-stained vomit in an infant is a sign of gut obstruction. In the neonate, it may indicate necrotising enterocolitis (NEC), particularly in a preterm infant. The timing of onset of symptoms makes NEC unlikely.
- The early onset of symptoms indicates a high gut obstruction.
- The triple bubble sign indicates a blockage beyond the duodenum and hence the jejunum. Multiple 'bubbles' may indicate ileal atresia.
- The bubbles are similar to fluid levels in older infants.

Examination tips

- Neonatal abdominal X-rays are common pictures in the examination, so practise and view as many as possible.
- Always check any 'plastic', i.e. endotracheal tubes, position of long lines, chest drains and particularly nasogastric tubes. These may be abnormal and the candidate *must not miss them* if they are abnormal.
- If there are structural gut anomalies, also review the upper gut (i.e. is there curling of the nasogastric tube in an oesophageal pouch?) the rectum (is there gas?); and the vertebrae for abnormality to exclude a syndrome such as the VATER/VACTERL syndrome.

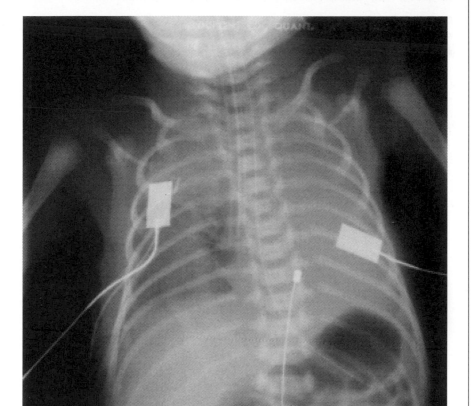

A 26-week gestation infant deteriorates during ventilation. A reintubation was performed without significant improvement in blood gases or oxygen saturation.

What abnormality is shown?

ANSWER 6

Misplaced endotracheal tube – situated in the right main bronchus.

Comments

- Always check for the position of various tubes, e.g. endotracheal tubes.
- Positioning of the endotracheal tube is critical – malpositioning is usually into the right main bronchus and often manifests as increased shadowing of the right upper lobe and the left lung due to collapse.
- Failure to interpret such an X-ray may result in a pneumothorax and therefore increased morbidity, particularly intraventricular haemorrhage, in the preterm neonate.

Examination tips

- Train yourself to look for iatrogenic issues on the X-ray such as the position of the endotracheal tube before returning to the area of interest or the obvious abnormality. This will avoid nasty surprises both in the exam and in clinical life!

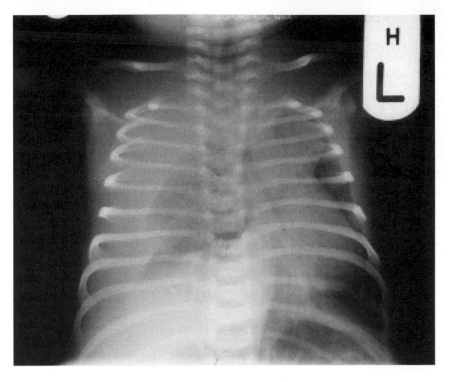

This chest X-ray was performed on a 2-day-old infant born after a normal delivery at term who was discharged home at 6 hours of age. Mother noted that the baby was feeding poorly and called the midwife who detected an elevated respiratory rate and grunting.

a) Describe the most significant radiological abnormality.
b) List two potential differential diagnoses.
c) Give one investigation to confirm your diagnosis.

ANSWER 7

a) Right-sided pleural collection with mediastinal shift.
b) Right chylothorax.
   Right pleural effusion.
   Right haemothorax.
   Right pyothorax/empyema.
c) Pleural tap and analysis of fluid.

Comments

- The radiological appearance of a pleural collection differs depending on whether the film is taken with the infant supine or held erect.
- When supine, the fluid is imaged beneath the lung, therefore increasing the density of the affected side.
- Usually the top of the fluid is seen sharply against the edge of the lung, providing the marked outline of the lung tissue as shown in this case.
- In the newborn the most likely cause of an isolated right-sided pleural collection is a chylothorax.
- Chylothoraces may result from:
   — trauma to the thoracic duct, e.g. post-thoracotomy, after chest drain insertion
   — spontaneous occurrence
   — congenital abnormality of the thoracic duct or lymphatics (pulmonary lymphangiectasia)
   — generalised lymphangiectasia.
- The cause and type of the collection are not determinable from the plain X-ray.
- Haemothoraces may occur as part of vitamin K-deficient haemorrhagic disease of the newborn.
- Congenital pneumonia may also produce a sympathetic effusion which can progress to an empyema. A chest ultrasound may demonstrate loculation in an organising empyema.
- Pleural fluid may occasionally contain fluid from total parenteral nutrition if the long line has migrated into the pulmonary vasculature and ruptured into the pleural, vascular and bronchial spaces.
- Analysis of the fluid obtained from a pleural tap will often be diagnostic and therefore is the preferable answer here rather than further imaging studies.

Examination tips

- This is a classic radiological appearance in clinical practice.
- The definite diagnosis cannot be specified from the X-ray, although cause may be inferred from an absence of clues, e.g. pneumonia, abnormally sited long line or abnormal clotting, either from the film or from the accompanying clinical history.

PASS ✓

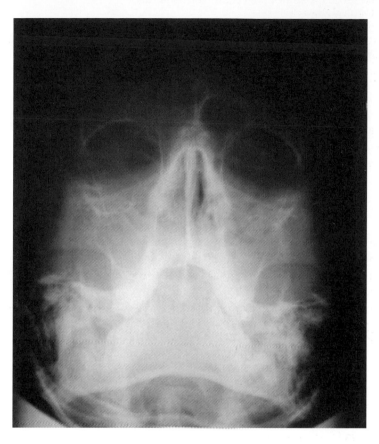

This teenage boy presented with a fever and headache but without evidence of a rash. Clinical examination confirmed evidence of pharyngitis and no meningism. However, his severe headache was sufficient to confine him to bed. His C-reactive protein level was 185 mg/L.

a) What radiological feature is demonstrated?
b) What is the diagnosis?

ANSWER 8

a) Fluid level apparent in the right frontal sinus.
b) Frontal sinusitis.

Comments

- The history indicates a probable bacterial infection but is not really indicative of meningitis. With headache a prominent feature, a sinus film has been performed which indicates a fluid level.
- Studies have shown that the most specific radiological sign of sinus infection is a fluid level. Clouding or increased opacity of a sinus does not appear as specific for infection as a fluid level.
- Remember that the frontal sinuses only become aerated and developed in the latter stages of childhood.
- Usually sinusitis is associated with other signs of an upper respiratory tract infection and is most commonly a clinical diagnosis.
- Sinus disease is best seen on CT scan.

Examination tips

- When faced with a film which is unfamiliar due to either position or type, keep to common principles such as comparing sides for symmetry etc.
- It is suggested that the following is a useful approach when the answer is not immediately apparent:

  P – check for 'plastic', i.e. tubes
  P – check whether a procedure has been performed
  C – check the corners of the field of interest
  C – check the corners of the X-ray film to ensure vital clues are not missed
  C – check for common problems
  P – now you may panic if you wish.

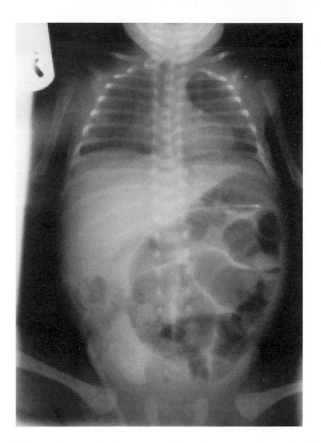

This is an abdominal X-ray of a 30-week gestation infant who has become unwell over the last 12 hours. Which of the following statements most closely fits your diagnosis.

a) The film indicates acute intussusception because of the paucity of right iliac fossa gas.

b) The film indicates malrotation because of the paucity of right iliac fossa gas.

c) The film indicates acute volvulus because of the predominantly left-sided gas patterns.

d) The film indicates a right iliac fossa tumour.

e) The film indicates necrotising enterocolitis with a right iliac fossa inflammatory mass.

ANSWER 9

The best answer is **(e)**.

Comments

- While the gas distribution is unusual, there is no evidence of either malrotation or volvulus.
- Necrotising enterocolitis is most likely based on the history.
- The right iliac fossa inflammatory mass is composed of loops of bowel matted together with oedema.
- Other radiological features of necrotising enterocolitis include:
  — distension of bowel loops
  — pneumatosis intestinalis
  — oedema of bowel wall
  — 'sick looking loops' – featureless sausage-shaped loops which persist on successive films
  — portal system gas (best seen over the lower margin of the liver shadow)
  — evidence of visceral perforation
  — abdominal wall oedema (not specific finding).

Examination tips

- As in this book, as in the exam – necrotising enterocolitis features quite highly in cases and it has several seemingly different presentations, as in this case.
- Always check for evidence of visceral perforation.

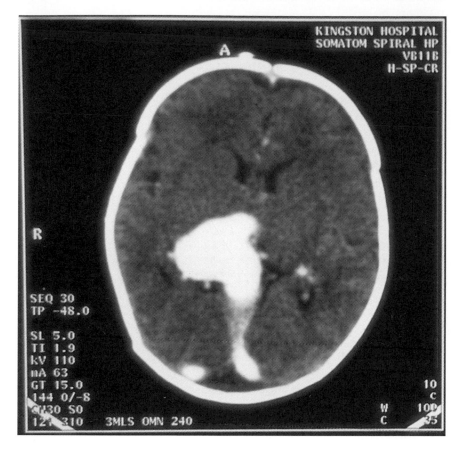

This is a CT with contrast brain scan of a newborn infant with cardiac failure. The chest X-ray and electrocardiogram were both normal.

a) What is the diagnosis?
b) What physical sign may develop or be present?
c) What is the treatment?
d) What complication may arise from (i) the disorder and (ii) the treatment?

ANSWER 10

a) Vein of Galen aneurysmal malformation.
b) Cranial bruit.
c) Selective embolisation.
d) (i) Shrinking brain (encephalomalacia) syndrome.
  (ii) Neurological deficits.

Comments

- When cardiac failure occurs in the newborn without evidence of obvious cardiac disease, always consider:
  — cardiomyopathy
  — total anomalous pulmonary venous drainage
  — intracranial arteriovenous or other vascular malformation
  — neonatal thyrotoxicosis.
- Vein of Galen aneurysmal malformation is a congenital vascular anomaly.
- The vein is usually a tiny short connection between deeper veins and draining sinuses.
- It is a rare anomaly.
- Detection may be antenatal where it is seen as an intracranial 'cyst'.
- Unsuspected occurrence usually presents with cardiac failure at about 48 hours of age.
- A bruit may not be present at delivery.
- The vascular nature of the lesion may be determined on ultrasound scan by the presence of bright echoes flashing across the lesion when microbubbles are introduced by the rapid flushing of a peripheral venous line with a saline flush.
- Untreated disease may result in encephalomalacia probably as a result of the pressure effect of the aneurysm.
- Current treatment involves embolisation of the lesion and not neuro-surgery.

Examination tips

- Remember to read the question – this is not blood but contrast as stated in the question.
- Contrast enhancement in this distribution indicates a vascular lesion.
- Some diagnoses are rare – note them down!

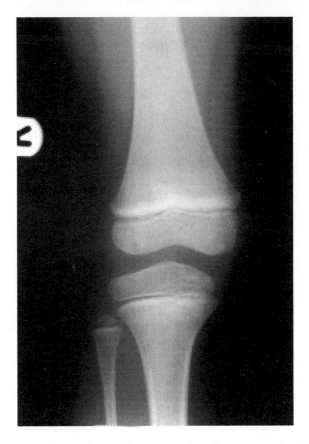

This X-ray was performed at a clinic visit. The boy was being investigated for unexplained hypochromic microcytic anaemia. He is known to have communication and behavioural problems.

a) What radiological abnormality is demonstrated?
b) What is the relationship of this abnormality to his anaemia?
c) Give two management strategies to treat this boy.

ANSWER 11

a) Radio dense line at the metaphyseal/epiphyseal junction ('lead lines').
b) Lead poisoning causing anaemia.
c) Avoidance of environmental cause and pica.
   Environmental investigation of source of lead.
   Treatment of lead toxicity including oral chelation with succimer or intravenous chelation in more serious cases with EDTA.
   Supportive therapy including admission to intensive care if encephalopathic.

Comments

- The most common source of lead remains lead-containing paints, particularly in properties built before the late 1950s.
- Lead poisoning remains a cause of acute encephalopathy.
- The diagnosis involves evidence of anaemia (which may be sideroblastic), basophil stippling on blood film, radiological evidence and elevated lead levels. Some authorities advocate analysis of porphyrin precursors of haem synthesis.
- Abdominal X-rays should be reviewed prior to chelation as lead flakes in the gut may be absorbed during chelation, therefore temporarily worsening the poisoning.
- Removal of source remains crucial.
- Repeated course of chelation may be necesssary.
- Chelation may also affect other trace metals such as copper and zinc so that supplementation may be necessary.

Examination tips

- This topic remains a popular one in the examination and in pre-examination courses.
- The lead lines are symmetrical.
- Check the blood film and the blood indices if available in the question.
- *Pica* = the ingestion of materials not usually considered to be a food.

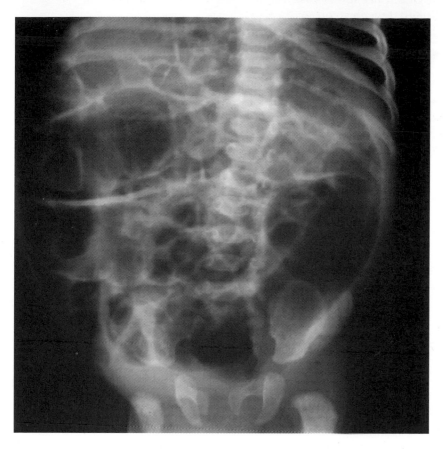

An infant was seen in clinic with a history of failure to thrive. Examination revealed abdominal distension. This abdominal X-ray was obtained.

a) What is the most likely diagnosis?
b) List one further investigation to aid diagnosis.

ANSWER 12

a) Hirschsprung's disease.
b) Rectal suction biopsy.

Comments

- The film shows dilated loops of bowel which is so marked that loops appear to be outside the body (obviously they are not!). There is a paucity of gas lower down in the bowel.
- The underlying pathology is a caudal absence of gastrointestinal wall nerve plexuses which may be determined by rectal suction biopsy. Occasionally, surgical full-thickness biopsies may be necessary.
- The classic history of delay in the passage of meconium is often absent. Usually symptoms occur at an early age, although some authorities state that later-onset disease may occur.
- Hirschsprung's disease may present with atypical neonatal necrotising enterocolitis in the older neonate.
- Management depends on the extent of the disease but is often surgical in nature.

Examination tips

- With apparent neonatal abdominal X-rays, always check:
  — where are the iatrogenic shadows of nasogastric tubes, drains, central lines, dye etc.
  — are there signs of NEC?
  — is there obstruction ?
  — are there abnormalities in the corners of the abdomen, e.g. peritoneal calcification after meconium peritonitis or evidence of free gas within the peritoneum?
  — is the abdominal wall thickened with oedema (as seen in major inflammatory conditions)?

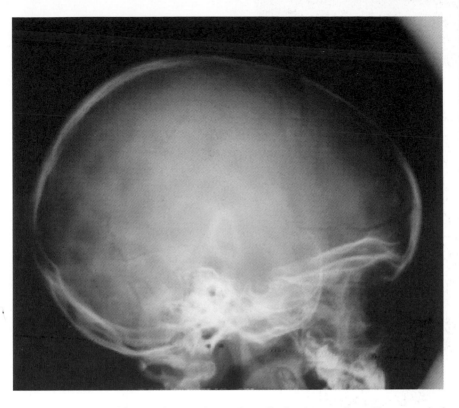

A 4-month-old child was dropped accidentally by his mother. She attended the A & E department immediately. On examination there was a large right frontal haematoma but the baby was otherwise neurologically normal. Which of the following statements most closely matches your subsequent assessment?

a) The linear fracture is indicative of non-accidental injury because it is straight-lined.
b) The linear fracture is not indicative of non-accidental injury because it is straight.
c) The linear fracture is indicative of non-accidental injury because skull fractures are rare in this age group of infants.
d) The linear fracture is not indicative of non-accidental injury because it is single and less than 5 mm in width.
e) The linear fracture is indicative of non-accidental injury because it is frontal in position.

ANSWER 13

The best answer is **(d)**.

Comments

- Skull fractures are relatively common in children.
- Skull fractures occur in falls from all heights but studies suggest that less than 2% of children falling from 4 feet (from adult waist height) suffer a fracture, probably as a result of protective reflexes or deflection of another presenting body part. Other studies have shown that the majority of still-born infants will suffer fractures from heights as little as 18 inches – presumably because of the loss of protective reflexes.
- The degree of injury also depends on the surface upon which contact occurs.
- In the infant, the head is significantly larger in proportion to the body than in adults.
- Single linear fractures (usually parietal) have low specificity for child abuse. An occipital fracture is more suspicious as greater force is necessary to sustain trauma via this thicker occipital bone.
- Narrow fractures are less suspicious of non-accidental injury, as in this case. Measurements exceeding 5 mm are classed as wide fractures.

Examination tips

- A skull X-ray may accompany a grey case or photographic section case pertaining to child abuse.
- The features indicating a suspicion of child abuse are a regular examination question in all paediatric examinations and may be the basis of a case discussion during the oral examination part of the MRCPCH.
- Skull fractures are notoriously difficult to identify – in the examination they will be significant if it is necessary to identify them.
- Always trace the outline of the whole of the skull outline in order not to miss a fracture or misinterpret a vascular shadow. A fracture will cross both bone tables. If in doubt, compare appearances of the same area in two planes, e.g. lateral and AP views.
- Remember that it is easier to visualize a fracture on the plain X-ray or CT scanogram rather than relying on the CT brain cuts themselves.

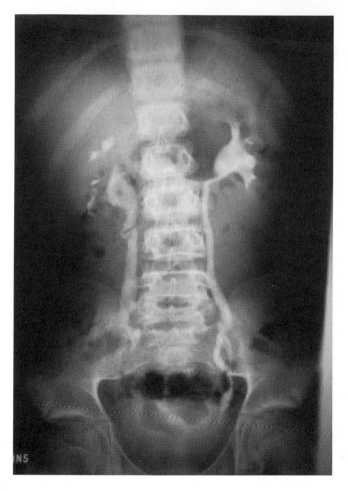

a) What investigation has been performed?
b) What abnormality has been demonstrated?
c) Give one further investigation to aid management.

ANSWER 14

a) Intravenous urogram.
b) Right megaureter.
c) DMSA or MAG3 radioisotope scan to determine renal function.

Comments

- A wide and tortuous ureter is suggestive of one of the following:
  — vesicoureteric reflux
  — obstruction at either the vesicoureteric junction or, if bilateral, the bladder outflow tract
  — congenital megaureter.
- These may be determined by a series of investigations to ensure the absence of reflux and the prompt excretion of dye, making a megaureter more likely than obstruction.
- A congenital megaureter may not need treatment and prophylaxis may only be necessary if urine infections coexist.

Examination tips

- Check for the appearance of the bladder and whether a catheter can be seen in order to determine whether this is an intravenous urogram or micturating cystourethrogram.
- Check for a renogram appearance.
- Check for renal or ureteric calculi which may coexist if renal disease is present or may even be the reason for the urogram in the first place.

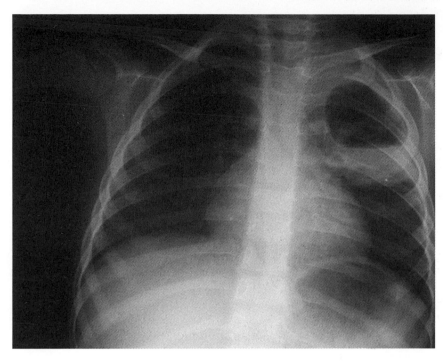

This child of 5 years of age was admitted with a rigor and fever. A respiratory rate of 40 breaths per minute was noted. This is the subsequent chest X-ray.

a) Give two differential diagnoses.
b) List two therapeutic manoeuvres to aid management.

ANSWER 15

a) Infected lung cyst (left).
Lung abscess.
Pneumatocele.
Cavitating lesion: pneumonia/tuberculous/aspergilloma.
b) Antibiotic therapy.
Physiotherapy.
Bronchoscopy.
Supportive care, e.g. oxygen.
Left upper lobectomy.

Comments

- There is a large left upper zone lesion containing an air–fluid level. The lesion appears thin-walled. This is most likely an infected lung cyst but an abscess cannot be completely excluded.
- The child is a little old for a staphylococcal pneumatocele, particularly as there is no history of immunodeficiency given. There is little surrounding evidence of a pneumonia to support the possibility of pneumonic cavitation.
- Tuberculous cavitation is unusual in children. This is not the typical appearance of an aspergilloma where there is usually a halo appearance of the fungal infection within the cyst.
- Treatment is usually antibiotics with supportive care. Further investigations such as a CT scan may be of benefit to delineate the aetiology of the lesion. Failure to respond or resolve will necessitate bronchoscopy. If the lesion is a congenital cyst then surgical resection may be necessary.

Examination tips

- Chest fluid levels occur in :
  — abscesses
  — infected cysts
  — unusual cysts, e.g. hydatid cyst
  — cavitating tumours (rare)
  — cavitating pneumonia
  — congenital diaphragmatic hernia.
- Write down your investigations or treatment options in a list of either the best options or the most diagnostic and therefore specific for your previously given diagnoses.

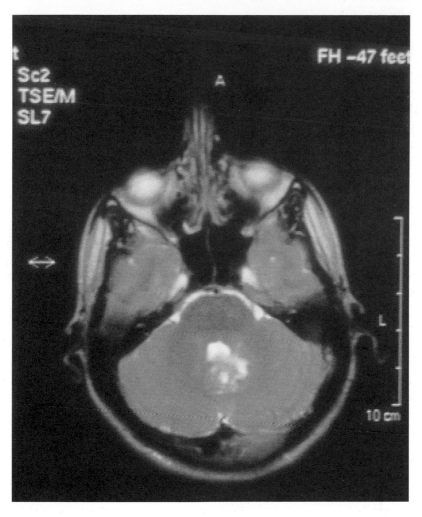

This central nervous system image was performed in a 3-year-old child with a headache and intermittent ataxia.

a) What abnormality is shown?
b) What is the worst prognosis lesion?
c) What is the differential diagnosis?

ANSWER 16

a) Posterior fossa space-occupying lesion in the cerebellar vermis extending into the cerebellar hemisphere.
b) Medulloblastoma.
c) Astrocytoma.
   Ependymoma.
   Cerebellar abscess.
   Hamartoma.

Comments

- An obvious space-occupying lesion presenting subacutely in this age group is likely to be a medulloblastoma.
- Medulloblastoma, a neural crest-derived tumour, is likely to metastasise early in the disease.
- Treatment is intensive, involving surgery, chemotherapy and radiotherapy.
- Posterior fossa tumours may present with raised intracranial pressure due to hydrocephalus resulting from an obstructed fourth ventricle.
- The posterior fossa remains the most common site for a central nervous system tumour.
- MRI scanning has significant advantages over CT scanning of the posterior fossa.

Examination tips

- Always examine the posterior fossa closely to look for a tumour.
- Check for signs of mass effect – low-density areas surrounding the mass on CT scan.
- Also exclude a dilated ventricular system indicating early hydrocephalus.
- The nature of the appearance of the tumour may give clues to its aetiology, i.e. calcification may indicate slower growth of the tumour.

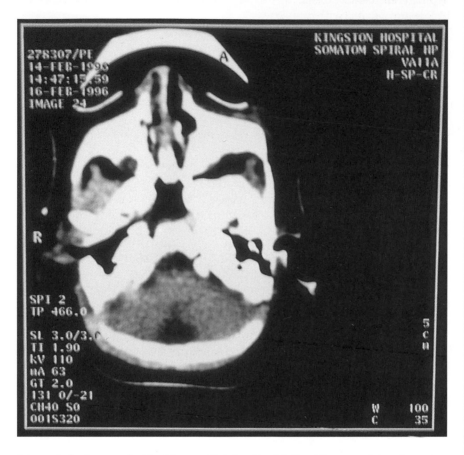

A term infant was admitted immediately after birth with unexplained respiratory distress. The chest X-ray and electrocardiogram were normal. An arterial blood gas revealed: pH 7.25, P_{CO_2} = 8.4 kPa, P_{O_2} = 5.1 kPa, HCO_3 = 17.2, BXs = -4.4. The illustrated investigation was performed.

a) What is the diagnosis?
b) What is the treatment?

ANSWER 17

a) Bilateral choanal atresia.
b) Supportive care with oral airway.
   Surgical correction with insertion of stents.
   Nasal toilet and the use of intranasal steroids.

Comments

- Upper airways obstruction is a comparatively rare cause of neonatal respiratory distress.
- Choanal atresia may be unilateral or bilateral.
- Choanal atresia may be isolated or syndromic, e.g. part of the CHARGE syndrome.
- The diagnosis may be suggested by difficulty in passing a nasogastric tube or by the prompt improvement of the infant's clinical state and blood gases when the obstruction is bypassed, such as after intubation when overventilation will occur despite minimal support.

Examination tips

- When a surprising or apparently irrelevant investigation is shown, check that your differential diagnosis is correct – it is rare that completely irrelevant investigations will be included in the photographic section.
- When presented with a radiological image of which you are unsure, compare sides and other views. This should make diagnoses like choanal atresia amenable to diagnosis.
- Occasionally the radiological appearance may include a nasal fluid level – do not be put off by this.

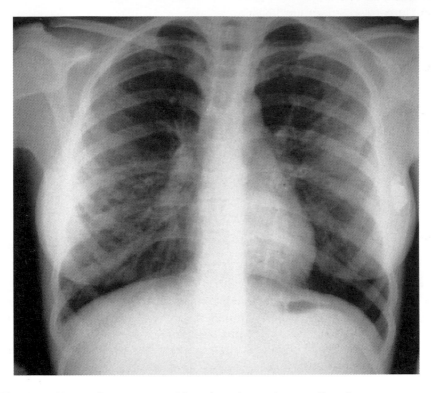

This is an X-ray of a teenager with a chronic respiratory disorder.

a) What is the most likely diagnosis?
b) Which of the following are typical radiological findings in this condition:
    i) cysts
    ii) linear atelectasis
    iii) ring shadows
    iv) bronchial wall thickening
    v) hilar lymphadenopathy?

ANSWER 18

a) Cystic fibrosis

b) The correct answers are: linear atelectasis
ring shadows
bronchial wall thickening.

Comments

- The cystic fibrosis chest X-ray is very variable and depends upon the age of the patient and the degree of illness.
- Characteristically, the X-ray shows areas of :
  — ring shadows – end on bronchi partially filled with pus and thickened lining
  — bronchial wall thickening – as above but linear
  — discrete area of atelectasis
  — areas of linear shadowing indicating bronchiectasis.
- Cysts rarely occur unless a pneumatocele occurs. Hilar lymphadenopathy may occur but this is not typical.
- The X-ray changes may be quantified by the Crispin Norman score which analyses various changes on both the PA and lateral chest films.

Examination tips

- Cystic fibrosis makes a regular appearance in the MRCPCH examination, thereby underlining its importance in clinical practice.
- An abnormal X-ray like this may well be part of a grey case.
- Haemoptysis may be a feature of the question and be used as the key to a question around cystic fibrosis.
- Remember the complications of cystic fibrosis, e.g. pseudo-Bartter's syndrome, meconium ileus equivalent, liver disease, diabetes, vasculitis and arthropathy.

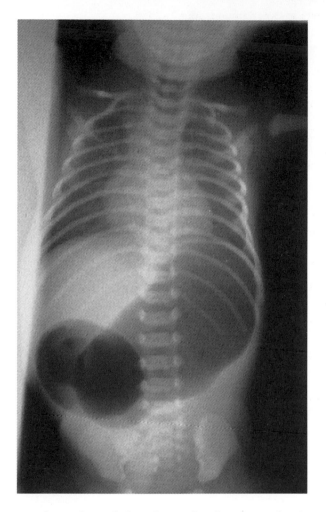

This film was performed on a baby admitted to the neonatal unit.

a) What is the diagnosis?
b) What else should be actively sought by:
   i) clinical examination
   ii) further investigation

ANSWER 19

a) Duodenal atresia.

b) i) Features of Down's syndrome.
   Cardiac abnormality, particularly atrioventricular septal defect.
   Gut atresia, e.g. imperforate anus.

   ii) Cardiac abnormality by echocardiogram.
   Hearing deficit by neonatal screening.

Comments

- The appearance is descriptively termed a 'double bubble', indicating high gut obstruction.
- Duodenal atresia may be associated with Down syndrome, as in this case.
- Whilst the cardiac silhouette and ECG will be of help, routine echocardiography remains the standard care.

Examination tips

- There are some diagnoses that must be recognised – this is one of them!

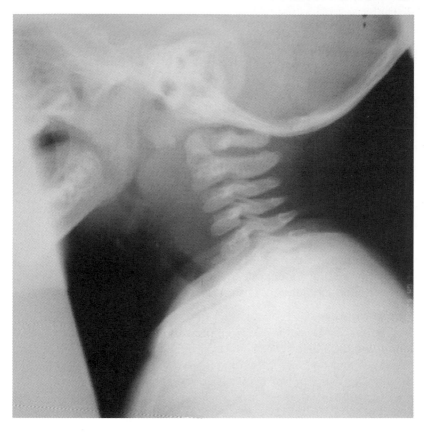

An infant was admitted with a mild fever and soft stridor. There was no evidence of shock and the child did not appear toxic. There was mild dysphagia.

a) What is the diagnosis?
b) Give two further investigations to aid the management of this patient.

ANSWER 20

a) Retropharyngeal oedema.
Retropharyngeal abscess.

b) CT or MRI of retropharyngeal space.
C-reactive protein – as a marker of infection.
Blood count and film – marker of sepsis.
Blood cultures.
ASO titre.

Comments

- The retropharyngeal space exceeds the normal space allowance – the width of the vertebral body. This indicates swelling. However, it is not possible to differentiate between oedema and an early abscess either radiologically or from the history.
- Always consider a foreign body.
- With the reduction in incidence of epiglottitis due to Hib vaccination, bacterial tracheitis ('bacterial croup') has become a more common entity and must be considered, as significant morbidity is attached to this diagnosis if appropriate treatment is not considered.
- Further imaging may identify pathology.
- Full resolution should occur with early antibiotic intervention.

Examination tips

- Despite the clinical reduction in epiglottitis, it must not be forgotten as a diagnosis either clinically or in the examination.
- The appearance radiologically of epiglottitis is one of discrete swelling of the epiglottis superior to the tracheal gas shadow.
- Always check for a radio-opaque foreign body

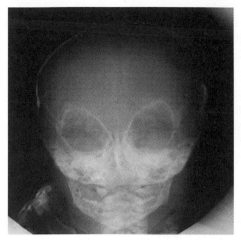
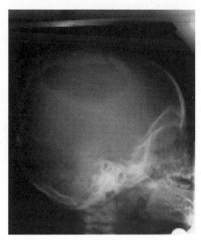

A   **B**

A 10-month-old infant suffered an accidental head injury with parietal skull fracture. Although initially lost to follow-up, the mother returned to clinic several weeks later. In view of her concerns and the clinical findings, a further skull X-ray was obtained.

a) What is the diagnosis?
b) What is the cause of this?
c) What is the treatment?

PASS

ANSWER 21

a) A growing fracture.
b) Leptomeningeal cyst.
c) Neurosurgical repair of the dural defect.

Comments

- A growing fracture is a widening defect in the skull after an initial fracture predominantly in the young infant. Clinically this child had an obvious pulsatile swelling over the fracture.
- The basic problem is a defect in the dura mater which is interspersed between the skull bones preventing closure and healing of the fracture. This is termed a leptomeningeal cyst which requires surgical repair.
- All infants below 2 years of age with a skull fracture require a follow-up appointment.

Examination tips

- Always check the two views of the skull before committing oneself to a diagnosis or description of abnormality.

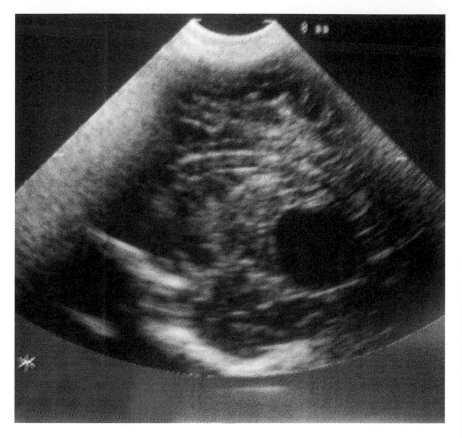

This is a neonatal cranial ultrasound scan.

a) What view is presented?
b) What abnormality is shown?
c) List two differential diagnoses of this abnormality.

ANSWER 22

a) Parasagittal view.
b) Intracranial cyst-like lesion.
c) Intracranial abscess.
   Vascular malformation, e.g. vein of Galen aneurysmal malformation.
   Arachnoid cyst.
   Porencephalic cyst.
   Primary developmental brain cyst.
   Primary neonatal brain tumour (very rare).

Comments

- A round black echo-poor area is seen inferiorly. This was vascular in origin and was a vein of Galen aneurysmal malformation (see Question 10).
- An arachnoid cyst is usually post-inflammatory and is an in-pocketing of the arachnoid meninges.
- Porencephalic cysts are usually large solitary areas which communicate with the ventricular system and arise after periventricular haemorrhage in the preterm infant. They are often superior to the lateral ventricle – hence this lesion is not in the expected location.

Examination tips

- Cranial ultrasound scans are appearing in the examination and examination texts more frequently. You must practise these as they are also commonly performed in most neonatal units. Paediatricians are often responsible for performing scans both routinely and in emergencies.
- Initially it is important to orientate oneself – this is a parasagittal view with the base of the skull appearing as a bright stepped line inferiorly and the nose at the left of the film. Ensure that you can distinguish between parasagittal and coronal views which are the most commonly used and displayed views.
- Check the film to see whether any clues are given to the side of the brain under investigation.
- Check the following:
   Ventricles – appearance, size, shape
   Evidence of a haemorrhage – size, side, extension and effect on ventricle
   Evidence of ventricular obstruction, e.g. visible IIIrd ventricle
   Choroid plexuses – any minor haemorrhage often occurs here
   Periventricular areas – for bright flares indicating potential ischaemic areas
   Scan anteriorly, posteriorly and laterally – ensure brain parenchyma is normal
   Midline view – identify the corpus callosum and septum pellucidum
   Coronal view – establish reproducibility of any abnormality seen already
   Coronal view – establish any midline shift.

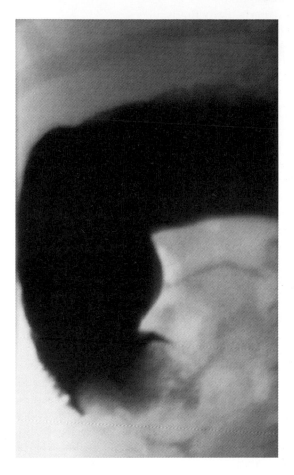

A child aged 18 months was admitted with a short history of bilious vomiting and abdominal pain. The child was poorly perfused although this responded to intravenous fluid replacement. The examination illustrated was performed.

a) What is the diagnosis?
b) What is the standard management of this disorder?

ANSWER 23

a) Acute intussusception.

b) Resuscitation, particularly fluids.

Analgesia and other supportive care.

Contrast or hydrostatic reduction if there are no contraindications to do so.

Surgical reduction if there are contraindications to the above or failure has occurred.

Comments

- This screening film identifies dye outlining both the intussusceptum and intusscipiens during attempted contrast reduction which has proceeded as far as the right iliac fossa.
- The plain X-ray may show a paucity of gas in the right iliac fossa (if it is the most common type of intussusception of ileocaecal origin) and dilated loops of proximal small bowel due to obstruction.
- The best course of action in such cases remains controversial – debate over which type of reduction continues in the literature.
- Contraindications to a non-surgical reduction include:
  — signs of perforation
  — peritonitis
  — poor clinical state
  — prolonged history
  — failure to sedate or massive sedative requirements
  — failure to reduce with standard reduction techniques.

Examination tips

- In view of the importance of this diagnosis, examples of acute intussusception are common on pre-examination courses and in the examination itself.
- When faced with contrast studies, try to follow the course of the dye in order to identify which type of contrast study has been performed, e.g. enema or meal. The latter will usually show evidence of the typical outline of the feathery small bowel lumen and not leave any remnants in the rectum. Often the film will be reduced down to the area of interest, as in this film.

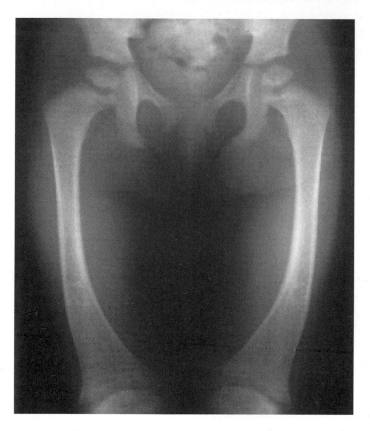

This X-ray was performed on a white Caucasian girl of 4 years who presented with gait difficulties where she was tripping over frequently. Her height was on the third centile. Her parents are not related by birth. Of note, mother mentioned that her daughter had suffered with a surprising amount of dental caries despite good oral hygiene. Subsequent investigations revealed a serum calcium of 2.43 mmol/L, alkaline phosphatase level of 235 IU/L and serum phosphate of 0.7 mmol/L.

a) What is the most likely diagnosis?
b) What is the appropriate treatment?
c) What is the inheritance pattern of your diagnosis?

ANSWER 24

a) X-linked hypophosphataemic rickets.
b) 1-alpha calcidol.
Oral phosphate supplements.
c) X-linked dominant.

Comments

- The X-ray shows typical features of rickets:
  — osteopenic bones
  — cupping/splaying of the metaphyses
  — bowing of the femora
  — irregularity of the metaphysial margin.
- The history also suggests a bone abnormality including the issue over stature and dental caries.
- The low serum phosphate in the presence of a normal calcium is suggestive of the diagnosis of hypophosphataemic rickets. The vitamin D level is usually normal.
- In view of its mode of inheritance, the presentation of disease is usually milder than in males.
- Treatment requires additional vitamin D and large doses of phosphate. Unfortunately the latter may result in diarrhoea. Normalisation of serum phosphate is associated with improved growth and both clinical and radiological straightening of the legs. However, long-term treatment may result in nephrocalcinosis – many authorities have linked the risk of nephrocalcinosis to the amount of phosphate required to treat the disorder.

Examination tips

- The appearance of rickets is rarely diagnostic and information should be sought from the question to aid definitive diagnosis and cause.

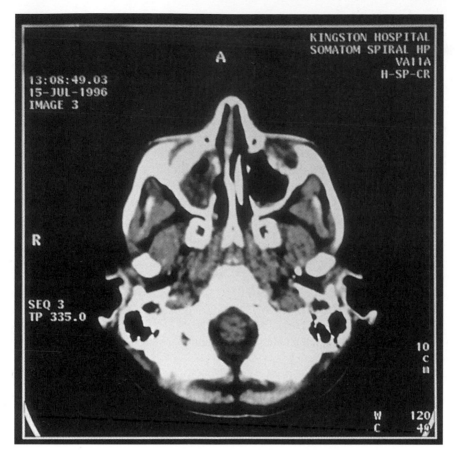

A CT scan was performed in a teenager with pneumococcal meningitis.

What is demonstrated?

ANSWER 25

Right maxillary sinusitis.

Comments

- Sinusitis is well demonstrated on CT scan.
- The risk of intracranial sepsis is increased with bacterial sinusitis because bacteria may be forced into the intracranial vaults as there is high pressure within the sinus space. The connecting veins are valveless, so bacteria may be deposited anywhere along these veins, including into the subarachnoid space, resulting in meningitis.
- Usually sinusitis is a clinical diagnosis.

Examination tips

- Again – if in doubt compare the two sides, having listed a potential differential diagnosis so that appropriate areas may be scrutinised. This will easily identify the opaque sinus antrum.

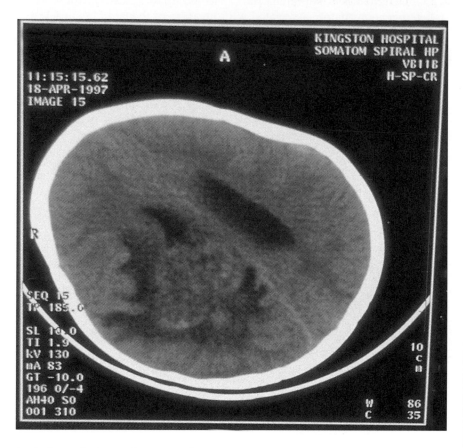

An infant of 12 months was referred to the clinic as there were concerns that his anterior fontanelle was large and his head circumference was above the 97th centile. The following scan was obtained.

a) Describe the abnormality.
b) Give the two most likely differential diagnoses.

ANSWER 26

a) Large right-sided supratentorial space-occupying lesion (tumour) of heterogeneous nature associated with invasion of the lateral ventricle and showing some mass effect or oedema.

b) Choroid plexus tumour.

Ependymoma.

Comments

- This tumour would appear to arise from the tissue surrounding the posterior part of the lateral ventricle and is encroaching on this structure. This is the site of the choroid plexus. The cells lining the ventricle may also be the source, e.g. ependymal cells. The heterogeneous nature of the lesion suggests that it is not a swiftly growing aggressive tumour, e.g. glioblastoma. There is some effect on the ventricles.
- Although macrocephaly is usually familial, other sinister causes need exclusion if there are associated symptoms or signs or an absence of other affected family members.
- Subsequent post-surgical epilepsy is well recognised as well as neuro-behavioural abnormalities.
- In this case, the tumour was of choroid plexus origin.

Examination tips

- In the presence of a brain tumour, ensure that the question does not indicate a neurocutaneous syndrome such as **tuberose sclerosis or neurofibromatosis type 1**, both of which are common in all parts of the examination and are commonly associated with central nervous system tumours.

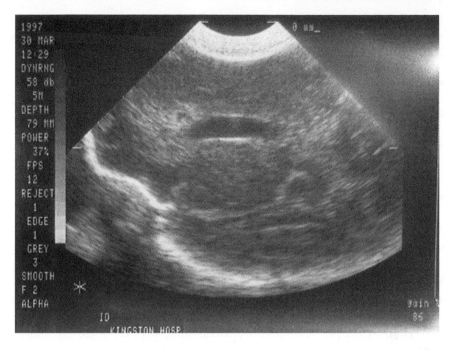

An ex-30-week gestation infant underwent a neonatal cranial ultrasound scan 4 weeks after birth. The delivery had been complicated by severe acidosis and hypotension. Respiratory support had been required for 1 week during which acute tubular necrosis had occurred. Which one statement accurately describes the scan appearance?

a) Small anterior cysts have developed indicating post-ischaemic periventricular leucomalacia.
b) Small anterior haemorrhage persists indicating periventricular leucomalacia.
c) Small anterior cysts have developed indicating post-haemorrhagic porencephaly.
d) Small anterior haemorrhage persists indicating the development of porencephaly.
e) Small anterior ischaemic flares persist.

ANSWER 27

The best answer is **(a)**.

Comments

- The appearance indicates the development of post-ischaemic cysts in the anterior region. These are separate from the ventricle and result from brain parenchymal necrosis.
- The ischaemic nature of these may be surmised from the history that was provided.
- The position of the lesions determines the potential subsequent neurological deficit – in this case a unilateral hemiparesis affecting mainly the arm.
- The cystic degeneration does not occur immediately so review scans are recommended where a risk of periventricular leucomalacia (PVL) is high. Early abnormalities on scans may be overlooked.
- PVL occurring in the first few days of life may indicate antenatal ischaemic lesions.
- Flares are bright echoes which may progress to cavitations in some cases but resolve in others. They are often periventricular or at 'watershed' areas between arterial supplies.

Examination tips

- Orientation of the scan and correct interpretation of additional history are important.
- Be able to differentiate between porencephaly and PVL.

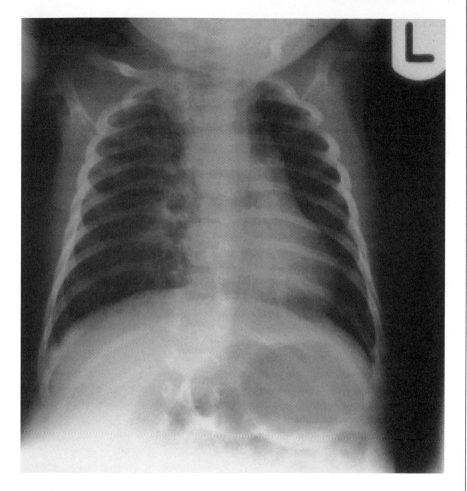

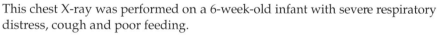

This chest X-ray was performed on a 6-week-old infant with severe respiratory distress, cough and poor feeding.

a) What is the most likely diagnosis?
b) List four other risk factors for severe disease.
c) What evidence-based therapies are recommended for treatment?

ANSWER 28

a) Acute bronchiolitis.
b) Chronic lung disease, e.g. cystic fibrosis or ex-preterm chronic lung disease.
   Congenital heart disease.
   Neuromuscular disease.
   Preterm infant.
   Metabolic disorder.
   Below 6 weeks of age.
   Immunodeficiency states.
c) Controversial and hotly debated (!), but probably only oxygen, if necessary, and good supportive medical and nursing care particularly with reference to feeding and hydration.

Comments

- The X-ray shows bilateral hyperinflation without focal abnormality (the 'ring shadow' is an artefact). The hyperinflation is due to air trapping similar to asthma. The history is suggestive of acute bronchiolitis.
- RSV (respiratory syncytial virus) remains the most common causative virus in epidemic acute bronchiolitis.
- In young infants, bronchiolitis may present with apnoea.
- Those with risk factors require special observation.
- Despite many studies, no completely effective therapy apart from oxygen and supportive care has been determined. Various studies examining the role of bronchodilators, steroids, adrenaline and the antiviral ribavirin have yielded varying results.
- Severe or atypical RSV infection may be the presenting feature of cystic fibrosis.
- Bronchiolitis-like infection may be the presenting feature of HIV infection.
- Approximately 5–8% of infants with RSV bronchiolitis may be coinfected with a bacterial infection.

Examination tips

- Remember to link an appropriate diagnosis with the correct age group, e.g. it would be unlikely for this to be asthma.
- When hyperinflation appears, ensure that it is not secondary to lobar collapse, e.g. right upper lobe – however, this is unlikely if it is bilateral.
- The liver may appear enlarged clinically but shown to be pushed down radiologically in bronchiolitis.

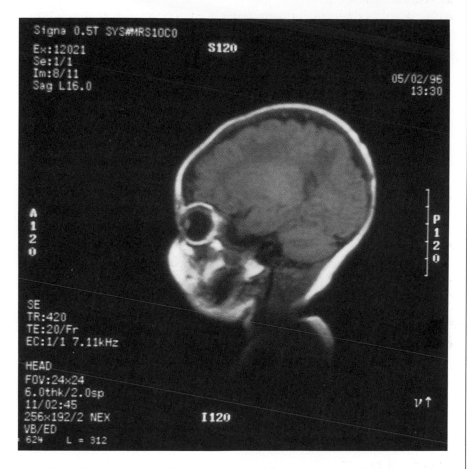

Signa 0.5T SYS#MRS10C0
Ex:12021
Se:1/1
Im:8/11
Sag L16.0

S120

05/02/96
13:30

A
1
2
0

P
1
2
0

SE
TR:420
TE:20/Fr
EC:1/1 7.11kHz

HEAD
FOV:24x24
6.0thk/2.0sp
11/02:45
256x192/2 NEX
VB/ED
624   L = 312

I120

An infant, born at term after an uneventful pregnancy and delivery, was investigated for intractable generalised seizures. Clinically the infant was not dysmorphic and her head circumference was on the 10th centile with her weight on the 50th centile. This investigation was performed.

a) What abnormality is shown?
b) What is the most likely cause?
c) What is the prognosis?

ANSWER 29

a) Polymicrogyria.
b) Neuronal migrational disorder.
c) Poor in terms of seizure control, neurodevelopment and life expectancy.

Comments

- This is a reconstructed MRI scan.
- The overall microcephalic nature of the underlying brain is demonstrated with a significant apparent degree of cerebral atrophy.
- The surface of the brain is subdivided into many small underdeveloped gyri.
- The pathological nature of this is a neuronal migration disorder occurring most commonly in the first and second trimesters. Histologically, heterotropias are seen.
- The degree of myelination is best determined by MRI in everyday clinical practice.
- Whilst this may be a feature of both syndromes and metabolic diseases, it is often idiopathic.
- Most children are significantly affected by their disorder.

Examination tips

- MRI scans are difficult to interpret for all of us apart from specialists and therefore few have appeared in non-radiology examinations so far. Practise by reviewing as many as possible.
- Those appearing in the examination will have significant abnormalities such as this one.
- As well as looking for specific abnormalities, always allow a short period of time to gauge the overall nature of the film/scan – in this case the small size of the brain is the clue.

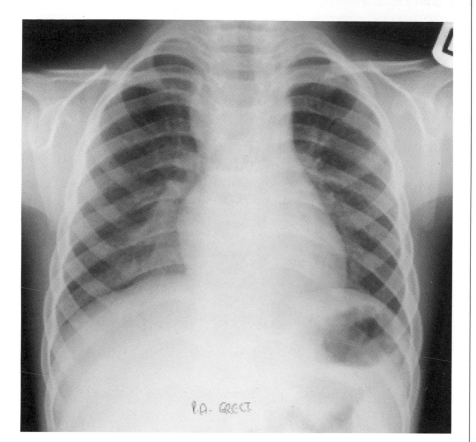

P.A. ERECT

This chest X-ray was reviewed. It had been requested for a patient who was uninjured in a road traffic accident. He had been wearing a safety belt.

a) What abnormality is demonstrated?
b) List three differential diagnoses accounting for this appearance.
c) What would be your next step in management provided the child remained perfectly well?

ANSWER 30

a) Mediastinal widening.
b) Damage to the aortic root.
   Thyroid abnormality.
   Thymus.
   Mediastinal lymph node disease, e.g. tuberculosis.
   Malignancy, e.g. lymphoma, teratoma.
   Bronchogenic cyst.
c) MRI thoracic inlet/mediastinum.
   Echocardiogram.

Comments

- The middle or anterior mediastinal widening is shown.
- The obvious concern relates to the history of trauma which increases the risk of aortic root damage. However, this was a thymoma.
- **Anterior mediastinal lesions** include:
  — thymus
  — thymoma
  — thyroid gland
  — teratoma
  — lymphoma.
- **Middle mediastinal disease:**
  — lymphoma
  — oesophageal diverticulum
  — tracheobronchial abnormalities
  — aortic disease
  — cardiac abnormalities, e.g. abnormal superior venous drainage in TAPVD.
- **Posterior mediastinal disease:**
  — neuroblastoma
  — ganglioneuroma
  — intrathoracic meningocele
  — neurenteric cyst.

Examination tips

- Do not forget to review the mediastinum as important disease may be present.
- Some questions may have more than one answer – provided that your answer is *consistent* with the lesion described or shown then it will attract some marks.
- Try to differentiate between the various layers of the mediastinum – the posterior mediastinal masses often have different radiological density from the others.

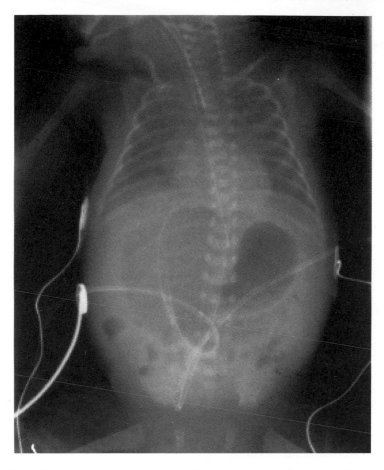

A 12-day-old preterm infant recovering from septicaemia suddenly deteriorated with discoloration of the anterior abdominal wall. This abdominal film was obtained urgently.

a) What radiological feature is shown?
b) What does this imply pathologically?
c) What is the diagnosis?

ANSWER 31

a) The 'football' sign – free gas manifest as a round 'football' lucency in the centre of the abdomen.
b) Visceral perforation.
c) Necrotising enterocolitis.

Comments

- The football sign is often accompanied by other signs of perforation, particularly the outlining of the falciform ligament in the centre of the abdomen.
- The free gas may be shown by a lateral shoot-through view, although this is rarely necessary in this situation.
- Deflation of the abdomen by the emergency introduction of an intra-abdominal cannula may be life-saving by reducing diaphragmatic splinting.
- Discoloration and oedema of the anterior abdominal wall are warning signs of impending or actual perforation.

Examination tips

- Do not ignore gas shadows which appear in a strange manner – they may indicate perforation.
- When one radiological feature of a particular disorder is noted, look diligently for others as in clinical life.

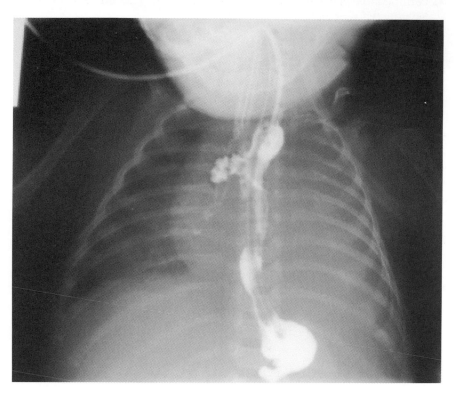

This infant underwent oesophagoscopy for presumed gastro-oesophageal reflux associated with recurrent respiratory symptoms. Subsequently the infant deteriorated with a fever postoperatively. A contrast study was performed.

a) Give two explanations for this appearance.
b) What is the probable cause of the fever?

ANSWER 32

a) Perioperative perforation of the oesophagus.
Existing 'H'-type tracheo-oesophageal fistula.
b) Mediastinitis.
Pneumonia.

Comments

- Contrast may be seen passing through a narrow aperture into the mediastinum. Contrast outlines the bronchial tree – this may be part of the fistula or as a result of regurgitation of dye and subsequent aspiration.
- 'H'-type fistulae are difficult to diagnose and often are only diagnosed by a combination of bronchoscopy/oesophagoscopy and radiological studies.
- There is some shadowing to suggest the onset of a lower respiratory tract infection.
- 'H'-type fistulae only account for approximately 5% of all tracheo-oesophageal fistulae.

Examination tips

- There is increasing emphasis on decision-making in the examination, i.e. what was the cause here rather than just pattern recognition or straight factual learning. Always balance the most likely scenario with the data/history provided.

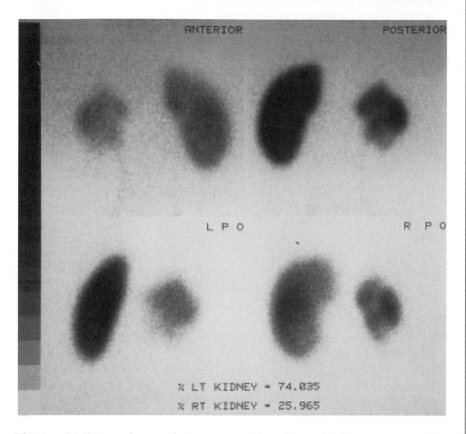

This is a DMSA renal scan of a teenager with mild renal failure as assessed by a slightly elevated serum creatinine. She has a history of possible urine infections as a child.

a) What is the interpretation of the scan?
b) What other investigation would be helpful to aid management?

ANSWER 33

a) Right renal scarring with reduced renal function probably as a result of earlier urinary tract infections.

b) Glomerular filtration rate (GFR).
Parathyroid hormone (PTH) estimation.
Wrist X-ray.

Comments

- The isotope film shows a right damaged kidney resulting in renal impairment.
- Frequent reflux of infected urine remains the most likely cause. A GFR will be most helpful to chart the degree of renal impairment.
- The PTH level and X-ray will allow an estimate of the degree of renal osteodystrophy to be made.
- The DMSA scan will identify even small amounts of scarring.
- Beware of a scan too soon after an infection where renal hypoperfusion may be mistaken for persistent scarring.
- The DMSA scan will give an accurate measurement of split renal function.

Examination tips

- These forms of isotope scans are becoming more popular in the examination.
- It may be difficult to differentiate between the scarred kidney and the dysplastic kidney.
- It is most likely that a DMSA wil be part of a more general question or a part of the data section.
- It is important to differentiate the DMSA and DTPA scan appearances and the data which may be derived from them.

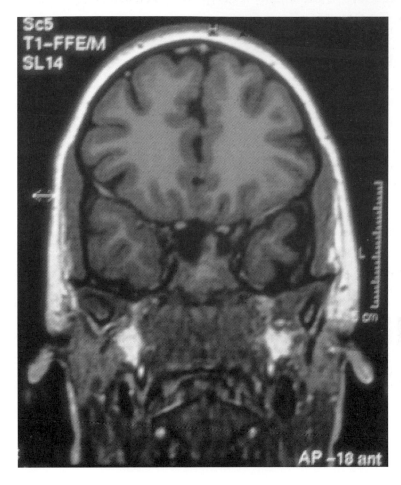

This cranial MRI scan was performed on a young girl with episodes of shaking and pallor during which she was completely aware. She suffered from pneumococcal meningitis at the age of 14 months.

a) What is the most likely diagnosis?
b) What is demonstrated on this MRI scan?
c) List three therapeutic interventions available.

ANSWER 34

a) Left temporal lobe atrophy with hippocampal sclerosis.
b) Partial epilepsy.
c) Anticonvulsants.
  Supportive therapy such as occupational therapy and educational support.
  Neurosurgery.

Comments

- The MRI shows considerable difference between the two sides.
- The history is suggestive of partial epilepsy or temporal lobe epilepsy.
- Hippocampal sclerosis may occur following meningitis or a prolonged febrile convulsion.
- Neurosurgical resection of damaged areas providing a focus for focal epilepsy is increasing in popularity.
- This child responded to carbamazepine monotherapy.
- Some of the newer anticonvulsants may also be of benefit as additional therapy for such disorders, e.g. lamotrigine.

Examination tips

- Thin slice MRI scans are the scan of choice for investigating hippocampal disease in children.
- Ensure that you are able to orientate yourself with the major MRI scans.

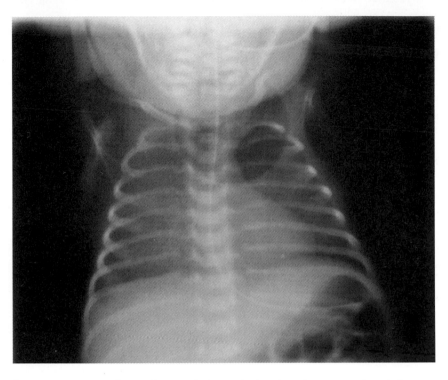

This X-ray was performed on an infant admitted to the neonatal unit because of hypoglycaemia and temperature instability. You are called to interpret the film.

a) What abnormality is shown?
b) What is the cause?

ANSWER 35

a) A circular radiolucent shadow over the lung field and right lung field shadowing suggestive of infection.

b) Artefact of the incubator roof hole appearing over the lung field!

Comments

- This film underlines the importance of not jumping to conclusions and studying all aspects of the film and the examination in question. Many artefacts are possible and they must be differentiated from true pathology.
- Always check whether any object overlies the area in question or is beneath it, e.g. hair clip in an older child etc.

Examination tips

- Although it would be unusual for a film to be included in the examination purely because of a 'trick', some films may include them as well as pathology so it is important to recognise them and thus avoid embarrassment.

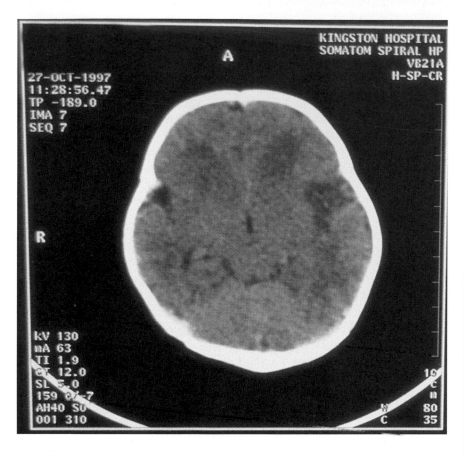

A newborn infant was admitted to the ward at 2 days of age having suffered a left focal seizure affecting her right arm predominantly. She was born after a Ventouse delivery but did not require admission to the neonatal unit. Examination was unremarkable and her fontanelle was soft. Further focal seizures were noted by the nursing staff.

a) This investigation was performed. What does it show?
b) Outline your further management of this infant.
c) What is the eventual neurological prognosis?

ANSWER 36

a) Left frontoparietal cerebral infarct.

b) Anticonvulsant therapy - traditionally phenobarbitone
Further investigation to ensure that there is no procoagulant tendency, e.g. protein S and protein C levels, homocystinuria screen etc.

c) Guarded, as various research papers quote differing risks – the most quoted is 8–10% risk of hemiplegia.

Comments

- The infarct is demonstrated as a low-density signal wedge appearing in the brain periphery. It is often, but not exclusively, in the territory of the middle cerebral artery.
- The appearance of the infarct will vary depending upon the timing of the scan.
- Many such infarcts are visible with ultrasound although some peripheral lesions may not be visible.
- MRI may confer some advantages.
- The precise timing is difficult and many are considered within the peri-delivery period.
- The incidence is higher in those undergoing an instrumental delivery, although an infarct may occur after a seemingly normal delivery.
- Rarely a procoagulant state is discovered. It may be that delivery does transiently increase the risk of infarction by increasing blood viscosity.
- The major risk is of hemiplegia. This may take several months to manifest.
- Follow-up ultrasound scans and CT may appear normal.
- A neonatal infarct may account for approximately 12% of all neonatal seizures.

Examination tips

- The appearance of the CT is usually diagnostic.
- Look for a wedge shape which is the most common presentation.
- This may be part of a larger question concerning the management of neonatal seizures or emergencies.
- Consider the timing of seizures as an aid to diagnosis of the underlying cause e.g.

Within 12 hours of delivery:
Cerebral malformations
Hypoxic encephalopathy
Hypoglycaemia
Intracranial haemorrhage

1–3 days post-delivery:
Metabolic disturbance such as hyponatraemia
Cerebral malformation
Drug withdrawal
Infection

4–7 days post-delivery:
Metabolic disorder
Infection
Hypocalcaemia

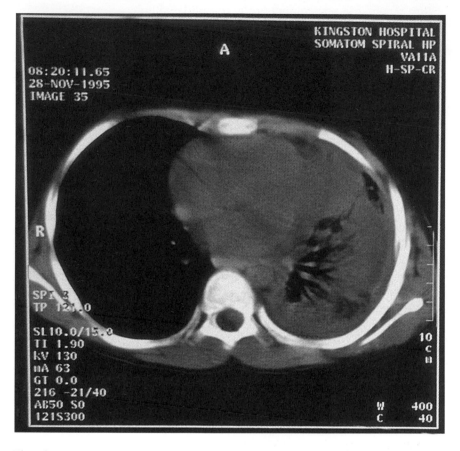

The above picture is a CT thorax scan. It was performed on a girl of 6 years with evidence of a severe left-sided pneumonia with persistent fever after 5 days of intravenous antibiotics.

a) List two radiological abnormalities.
b) What is the diagnosis?
c) What is the subsequent management of this problem?

ANSWER 37

a) Consolidated lung.
   Rim of solid tissue surrounding the consolidated lung.
b) Left empyema.
c) This remains controversial but at this stage surgical decortication is necessary.

Comments

- The scan demonstrates the thickened 'rind' of the empyema. In fact this had been demonstrated by chest X-ray and chest ultrasound scan. The CT was performed when closed chest drains failed to eradicate the empyema.
- The management of empyema is varied – many favour early chest drain insertion with the instillation of streptokinase to try to break down the developing loculations. Many children will improve spontaneously if the infection can be eradicated as measured by falling inflammatory markers and defervescence of fever. However, surgical stripping of the organised pus may be required despite early treatment with antibiotics and insertion of a chest drain.
- Some authorities suggest that any significant pleural effusion should be tapped as a diagnostic thoracocentesis to ensure that pus is not present – this procedure may need to be repeated depending upon the clinical progression.

Examination tips

- Unusual films may be included – the approach to these has already been suggested (answer 8).
- This example demonstrates how important it is to review the whole of the field in question. Otherwise it would be easy to miss the empyema.

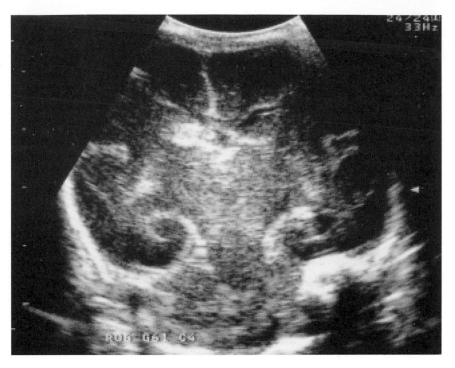

Which of the following statements regarding this neonatal cranial ultrasound scan is correct?

a) This is a parasagittal view demonstrating an anterior parenchymal flare.
b) This is a coronal section showing an anterior parenchymal flare.
c) This is a coronal section showing unilateral intraventricular haemorrhage.
d) This is a midline lateral view showing bilateral ventricular haemorrhage.
e) This is a sagittal view showing hydrocephalus and an anterior flare.

ANSWER 38

The best answer is **(c)**.

Comments

- This is a coronal section demonstrating the ventricles with evidence of haemorrhage. The ventricles are not dilated.
- There are several scoring schemes for intraventricular haemorrhage – therefore it is often better to describe what you can see.
- One standard score is:
  grade 1 – germinal matrix haemorrhage involving the ventricle
  grade 2 – haemorrhage involving the ventricle but not causing ventricular dilatation
  grade 3 – haemorrhage into the ventricle and causing dilatation of the ventricle
  grade 4 – haemorrhage extending into the surrounding brain parenchyma.
- Post-haemorrhagic ventricular dilatation is common, particularly after grade 3 and 4 haemorrhages.
- Ventricular dilatation may arrest and does not always progress onto progressive hydrocephalus requiring therapy.

Examination tips

- These scans are common so experience in their interpretation is necessary.
- The lesions should be obvious and usually are haemorrhages.
- Orientation and a knowledge of the different views (as in this question) are vital.
- Look particularly for bright rounded echoes within the ventricles (clots) and then any extension outside the ventricle into the surrounding brain.

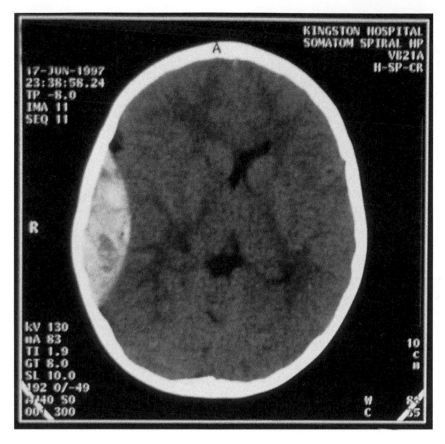

A 5-year-old boy was admitted to the resuscitation area having fallen off a swing. Although he seemed well initially, he became drowsy and vomited. On examination he has irregularly sized pupils which react to light. His Glasgow Coma Score is 8.

a) What is the diagnosis?
b) What is your management plan?

ANSWER 39

a) Right extradural haematoma.
b) Resuscitation with intubation.
   Urgent neurosurgical referral for craniotomy and removal of haematoma.

Comments

- The history is strongly suggestive of an extradural haemorrhage.
- The scan demonstrates the haemorrhage which characteristically bows into the brain tissue as the arterial bleed strips away the dura.
- The side of the lesion will be demonstrated by the abnormal pupil although bilateral abnormalities will occur as herniation of the brain becomes imminent.
- This is a neurosurgical emergency; however, good prompt resuscitation is vital – one study suggested that adverse outcomes in those with serious head injury could be reduced in 40% if resuscitation was effective, particularly in relation to the avoidance of hypoxia which will cause secondary brain injury if allowed to occur.
- The extradural is usually associated with a skull fracture through the middle cerebral artery.

Examination tips

- This is a classic case with a typical CT finding.
- Know your CT scan appearances of the extradural, subdural and sub-arachnoid haemorrhages:
  — **extradural:** high density with the collection bowing into the brain causing compression
  — **subdural:** variable density surrounding the brain but not bowing into it
  — **subarachnoid:** fresh high signal blood often outlining the falx.

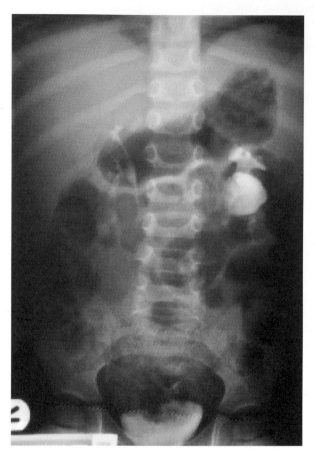

A child underwent a renal ultrasound scan as part of investigations of a urinary tract infection. A cyst-like structure was noted in the right kidney. This investigation was performed.

a) What investigation has been performed?
b) What is the most likely explanation for this appearance?

ANSWER 40

a) Intravenous urogram (IVU).
b) Left dilated calyx filling with dye and appearing as a cyst.

Comments

- The IVU will determine whether the cyst-like structure connects with the collecting system as it will become filled with dye. This excludes isolated renal cysts which may be:
  — congenital anomaly
  — malignant tumour.
- Although less frequently used, the IVU is of help in determining the structural appearance of some urinary tract abnormalities.
- In this circumstance, the cause is an isolated congenital abnormality of no significance.

Examination tips

- *Carefully check the following areas on an IVU:*
  — position of the calyces – to exclude a rotated kidney at risk of obstruction
  — the renal shadow, if present
  — position of kidney
  — dilatation of the calyces
  — tortuosity of the ureter
  — evidence of obstruction along the urinary tract
  — any difference between the sides
  — appearance of the bladder outline.

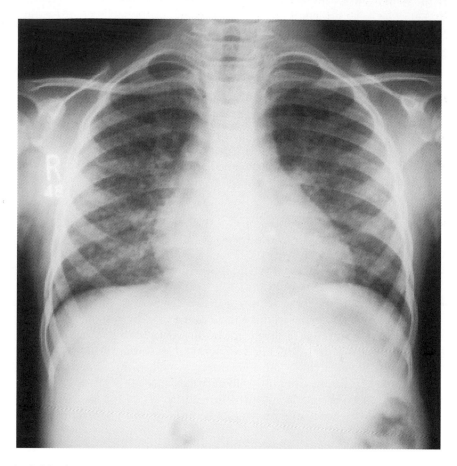

A child of 7 years was referred with breathlessness. She is the oldest child of refugee parents who have three younger children. She was noted to be losing weight and generally unwell. Her cough is non-productive.

a) Give two potential differential diagnoses.
b) List two investigations to aid diagnosis.
c) What additional investigations would you perform in this family?

ANSWER 41

Occasionally, there may be more than one potential answer. In this situation, decide which is the most likely. If a series of possibilities exists and investigations are requested, give the best (i.e. the most specific) answer to each of the differential diagnoses.

a) Miliary tuberculosis.
Lymphocytic interstitial pneumonitis (LIP).

b) Mantoux test.
HIV antibody assay.

c) Depending on the diagnosis:
Miliary tuberculosis – investigate other family members with chest X-rays and PPD (either Heaf or Mantoux tests). Isolate smear-positive adults when infected for the first 2 weeks of treatment if possible. Use chemo-prophylaxis where indicated.
Lymphocytic interstitial pneumonitis – investigate other siblings and parents for HIV status.

Comments

- The X-ray shows a bilateral reticulonodular appearance compatible with either TB or LIP.
- The history is compatible with either diagnosis. Statistically TB is the most common, with approximately one-third of the world's population infected. However, HIV infection is also of epidemic proportions.
- This film was, in fact, LIP. LIP is associated with the insidious onset of dyspnoea together with other features which include parotid gland enlargement. The cause of LIP is still debated.
- PPD tests may be falsely negative in miliary TB. A repeat test may be necessary. Evidence of other haematogenously spread TB infection should be sought.
- Be aware of the local and national guidelines (British Thoracic Society Guidelines 1998).

Examination tips

- TB may appear in all sorts of guises in the examination particularly:
  — TB meningitis
  — TB peritonitis
  — TB renal and bone disease
  — miliary TB.
- HIV remains a popular and common examination topic. It is well covered in many pre-examination courses and texts.
- Remember both diagnoses as part of many extensive differential diagnoses and therefore be aware of how to confirm the diagnosis as well as having an idea of treatment plans.
- With the exception of TB meningitis, the current guidelines suggest triple anti-TB therapy for 2 months (rifampicin, isoniazid and pyrazinamide) followed by dual therapy (rifampicin and isoniazid) for a further 4 months in the absence of multi-drug resistance.

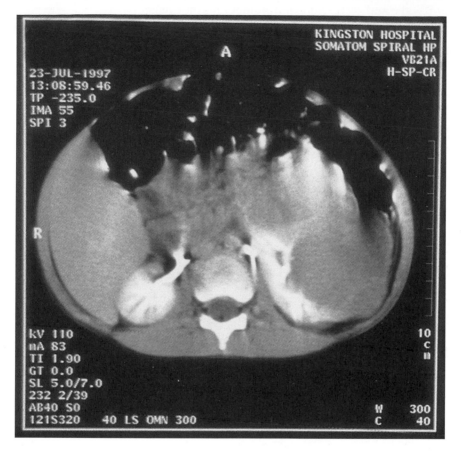

This abdominal CT scan was obtained in a child with a palpable abdominal mass. The child appeared well. Urinalysis was normal. The ESR was elevated at 25mm/hour. The blood pressure was 150/100 mmHg. His medical history was unremarkable with only a correction of a hypospadias of significance.

a) What is the most likely diagnosis?
b) Give three other important investigations to aid subsequent management.

ANSWER 42

a) Left Wilms' tumour.

b) Blood count – to exclude intratumour haemorrhage.
Serum electrolytes, urea and creatinine – estimate renal function.
Clotting studies – a von Willebrand type defect has been recorded.
Urinary catecholamine assays – to exclude neuroblastoma as a diagnosis.
Chest X-ray – to detect pulmonary metastases (occurring in 10% of cases); may use CT scan.
Biopsy and surgical staging.

Comments

- This is an embryonic neoplasm accounting for 8–10% of childhood malignancy.
- Few cases present after 11 years and most (90%) present before 7 years of age.
- Although there are associated predisposing conditions, the majority are sporadic.
- *Associated anomalies include:*
  - genitourinary abnormalities
  - hemihypertrophy
  - aniridia
  - Beckwith syndrome
  - WAGR complex (**W**ilms, **a**niridia, **g**onadal dysplasia and **r**etardation)
  - Denys Drash syndrome (Wilms, nephropathy and genital abnormalities).
- Calcification of the tumour occurs in less than 10% of cases (unlike neuroblastoma).
- Hypertension is a relatively rare occurrence but may occur as a result of excess renin, coexisting renal disease and vascular compression exerted by the tumour.
- Prognosis is related to stage and histology.
- Although most cases require surgery, the timing of surgery is debated. Preoperative chemotherapy may be used.

Examination tips

- Explore the site of origin of the mass and compare both sides.
- Wilms' tumours may have apparent blood pooling in them, manifest as low-density signal.
- Compare the history and radiological signs to distinguish between Wilms' tumour and neuroblastoma.

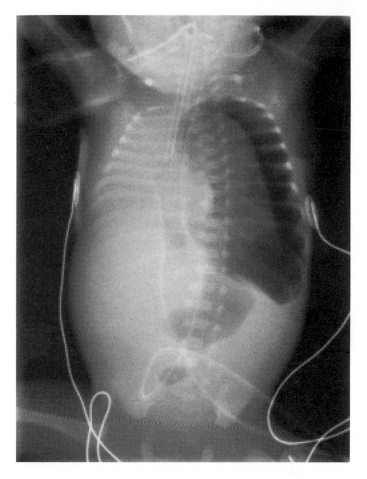

A preterm neonate was ventilated for respiratory failure. During ventilation there was clinical deterioration. The following blood gas was obtained: pH 7.22, P_{CO_2} = 8.9 kPa, P_{O_2} = 4.3 kPa, HCO_3 = 17.5 mmol/L, BXs = −4.5. The following chest X-ray was obtained.

a) What is the diagnosis?
b) What complication may occur?
c) How may you try to avoid this complication?

ANSWER 43

a) Left tension pneumothorax.
b) Periventricular haemorrhage.
   Bronchopleural fistula.
c) Avoidance of high ventilatory pressures.
   Avoidance of asynchronous ventilatory pattern.

Comments

- The presence of a pneumothorax is heralded by respiratory deterioration together with a worsening set of blood gases. This blood gas identified a worsening respiratory acidosis.
- Radiologically, the pneumothorax is a radiolucent shadow in the lung field. A tension pneumothorax is identified by its effect on its neighbouring structures, particularly causing mediastinal shift.
- The effect on cardiac output and cerebral perfusion followed by changes when the air leak is drained predispose to periventricular haemorrhage. The continuing presence of an air leak may indicate a bronchopleural fistula which is fortunately rare in clinical practice.
- Avoidance of risk factors includes avoidance of high mean airway and peak inspiratory pressures as well as ensuring synchronous ventilation using patient-triggered modalities, adequate sedation or, less frequently nowadays, artificial paralysis.

Examination tips

- Check the position of the mediastinum to ensure that there is no shift.
- Check whether there is evidence of previous pneumothoraces as demonstrated by the presence of indwelling chest drains – as always, look specifically for any foreign bodies.
- Exclude other air leaks such as a pneumomediastinum.

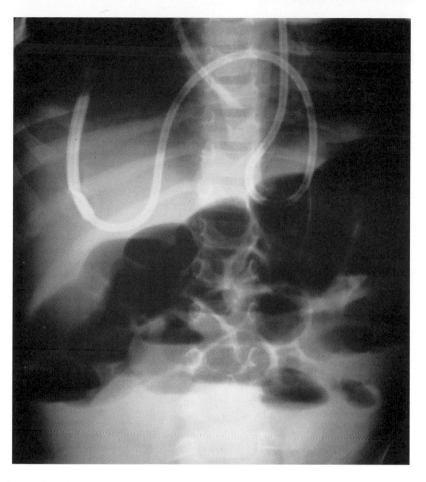

What is the diagnosis?

ANSWER 44

Small bowel obstruction.

Comments

- There are distended loops of bowel, particularly in the centre of the abdomen. The fluid levels on the erect film are strongly suggestive of bowel obstruction.
- *The most common causes of small bowel obstruction include:*
  — obstructed herniae
  — intussusception
  — malrotation
  — adhesions
  — volvulus.

Examination tips

- Sometimes the history will be suggestive particularly in the infant. Remember that bilious vomiting in infants below 18 months of age is strongly suggestive of obstructive gut disease.
- The appearance of haustrae may aid differentiation of large from small bowel obstruction, as may the actual distribution of the shadows.
- Check to see whether gas shadows are present in the area of the hernial orifices.

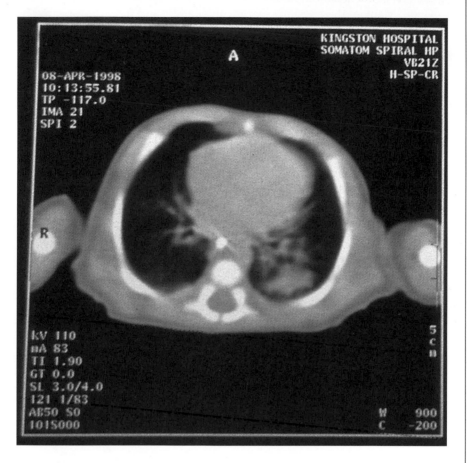

A CT thorax scan was obtained in a newborn infant who had been known to have an unusual thoracic appearance on antenatal scans. This is the postnatal CT scan.

a) What is the most likely diagnosis?
b) What is the prognosis?

ANSWER 45

a) Left cystic adenomatoid malformation.

b) Good. Many of these lesions regress antenatally and have disappeared by the time of delivery. Others resolve within the first year of life. Others, particularly large lesions, require surgical excision.

Comments

- Congenital lung cysts are a complex group of disorders. Cystic adeno- matoid malformation is one of the most important to be aware of.
- The lesion may be described in terms of the number and size of the cysts. It is believed that this may aid determination of the prognosis.
- Large lesions may be associated with antenatal polyhydramnios.
- Occasionally, very large lesions may compromise respiration at delivery.

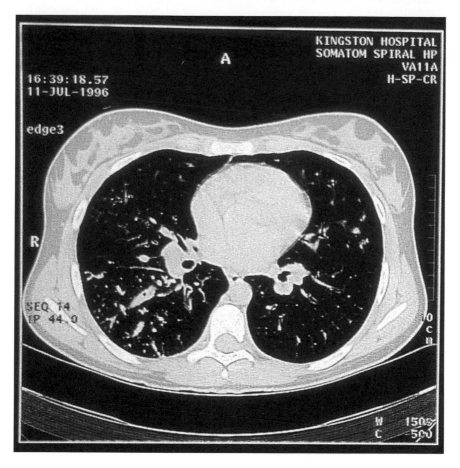

This boy presented to the A&E department with a large haemoptysis. He had a chronic non-productive cough. He did not require resuscitation and was haemodynamically stable. He subsequently suffered a further episode during his CT scan.

a) What is the diagnosis?
b) List three underlying differential diagnoses.
c) Outline your management.

ANSWER 46

a) Bilateral bronchiectasis.
b) Bronchiectasis following pertussis, measles or another severe lung infection.
   Primary ciliary dyskinesia.
   Cystic fibrosis.
c) Resuscitation if necessary.
   Antibiotics.
   Physiotherapy.
   Bronchoscopy.
   Surgical lobe resection.

Comments

- The scan demonstrates bilateral bronchiectasis with fluid containing shadows. As it is bilateral, the diagnoses of cystic fibrosis and ciliary dyskinesia are likely.
- Haemoptysis is most commonly associated with bronchiectasis.
- In this case, the cause was cystic fibrosis.
- Often, there is no immediate need for resuscitation after a haemoptysis.
- Severe bronchiectasis in one lobe may be cured by lobectomy.

Examination tips

- Bilateral disease is most likely to fit with the diagnosis of cystic fibrosis.
- The appearance may be severe or bilateral and only showing widened shadows in a tree-root distribution.
- The rest of the lung tissue is usually normal.

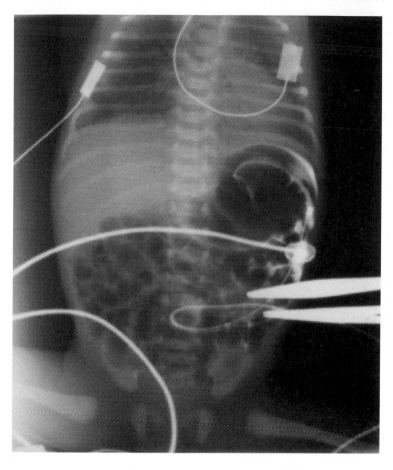

A preterm infant was admitted to the neonatal unit with respiratory distress. Intravenous fluids were commenced. An umbilical arterial line was inserted. In view of the failure of this line to sample satisfactorily, this film was performed.

a) What has been performed?
b) What is the explanation of this result?

PASS

Answer 47

ANSWER 47

a) Radio-opaque contrast has been injected down the umbilical arterial line.

b) The umbilical arterial line has ruptured into the peritoneal cavity. Contrast is seen collecting in the upper left abdominal cavity and outlining the stomach wall.

Comments

- Clinically, the interpretation of such films is important. Aberrant positioning of inserted lines is common and may be associated with a host of complications.

- Always be certain of the position of the tip of any inserted line, particularly when there are many other shadows present, e.g. around the thoracic inlet.

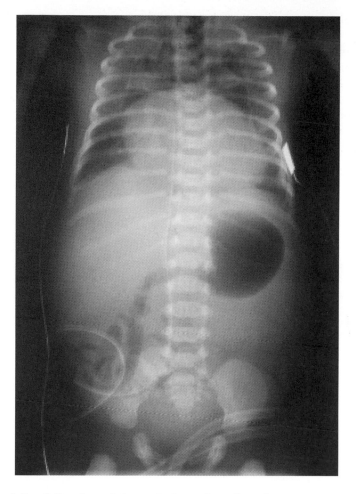

Which of the following statements best describes the appearance of this neonatal chest X-ray?

a) The lucent area above the heart represents a superior pneumo-mediastinum.
b) The lucent area above the heart represents a superior pneumothorax.
c) The lucent area above the heart represents a resolving pneumoperi-cardium.
d) The lucent area above the heart is a combination of pneumomediastinum and pneumopericardium
e) The lucent area above the heart is a radiological artefact.

ANSWER 48

The best answer is **(a)**.

Comments
- This is an unusual radiological appearance.
- The apparent loss of the superior pneumomediastinum is due to obscuring by collected air. It also gives the appearance of reducing the heart silhouette to that of an egg.
- This must be differentiated from the silhouette of cardiac defects, e.g. transposition of the great arteries (narrow superior mediastinum) or Fallot's tetralogy (apparent 'boot-shaped' heart with an elevated cardiac apex).

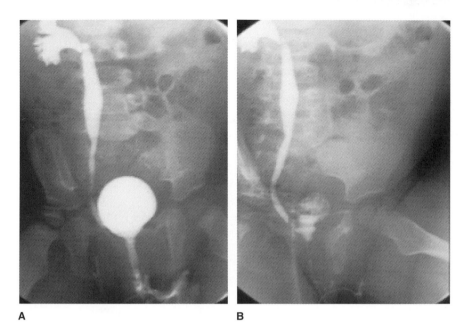

A   B

A girl of 9 months was referred for consideration of further investigation for renal abnormalities following her first documented urinary tract infection. A renal and bladder ultrasound scan suggested disparity in renal sizes.

a) What investigation is shown?
b) What is the diagnosis?
c) What other investigation may be of benefit and why?

ANSWER 49

a) Micturating cystourethrogram (MCUG).

b) Right vesicoureteric reflux up to the calyces but not distending them (grade IV).

c) DMSA radioisotope scan to determine split renal function and to determine whether the disparity between the kidney dimensions is due to renal scarring.

Comments

- This is an MCUG – this may be determined by both the appearance of the bladder outline and the presence of a catheter, which should be sought.
- Reflux may be described by a scoring system.
- Approximately one-third of children with a urinary tract infection occurring before 4 years of age may have vesicoureteric reflux. Many will suffer renal scarring, often occurring during the first infection.
- Most children will grow out of their reflux between 4 and 6 years of age. This has led to most children being managed with conservative antibiotic prophylaxis in the UK.
- Recurrent breakthrough infections despite adequate prophylaxis and compliance may necessitate ureteric implantation or other ureteric surgery to resolve the reflux.
- Renal scarring is a major risk factor for early hypertension.
- In older children, radioisotope scans such as DTPA scans may provide indirect reflux studies.

Examination tips

- Do not worry too much about learning scoring schemes – if they are forgotten in the heat of the examination, it is better to describe accurately and succinctly the abnormality and its severity.
- Ensure that you quote which side is affected.

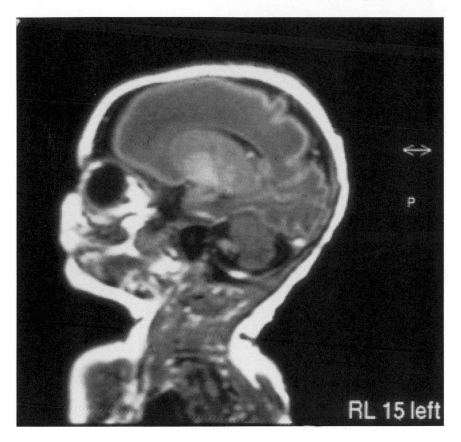

RL 15 left

A term infant weighing 3.7 kg was found apnoeic in his cot during a neonatal examination. On admission to the neonatal unit, he was found to be fitting. His biochemistry was normal and an infection screen, including cerebrospinal fluid analysis, was normal. A cranial ultrasound scan was reported as normal. This investigation was performed.

a) What investigation has been performed?
b) Describe the appearance of the cerebral cortex.
c) What is the diagnosis?

ANSWER 50

a) Cranial MRI scan.
b) Relatively smooth featureless cortex.
c) Pachygyria (lissencephaly).

Comments

- The cortex has fewer gyria than expected. This smooth surface is one of the variations of neuronal migration defects.
- Compare with Question 29.
- The prognosis of this group of lesions is generally poor in terms of both life expectancy and neurodevelopmental outcome.
- There is often associated cerebral atrophy.
- The head circumference may be normal or, more commonly, small.
- These lesions are rarely amenable to antenatal diagnosis. Although some may be features of syndromes or metabolic disorders, the majority are sporadic genetic in origin.

Examination tips

- Try to review cranial MRI scans in both sagittal and coronal views.
- Be aware of the different appearances of T1 and T2 weighted scans (T2 scans show up fluid as white, e.g. cerebrospinal fluid).

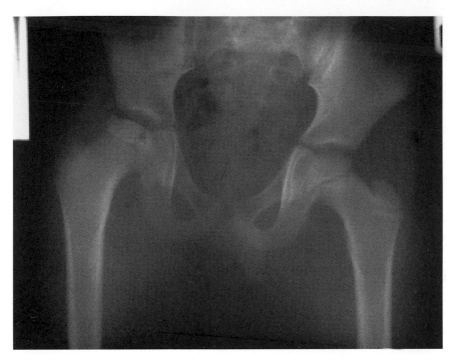

A 7-year-old boy was referred by his general practitioner with a mildly painful right knee causing him to limp. This X-ray was performed.

What is the diagnosis?

ANSWER 51

Right Perthes' disease.

Comments

- Perthes' disease may be unilateral or bilateral.
- It is generally not acutely painful and the pain may be localised to the ipsilateral knee or medial aspect of the ipsilateral thigh.
- The underlying pathology is an avascular necrosis of the femoral head.
- Aetiologically, Perthes' disease may be associated in some cases with preceding irritable hip where it is theorised that intra-articular pressure is raised thereby interrupting the vascular supply.
- Diagnosis may be suggested by limitation in movements of the hip, particularly external rotation, although all movements may be affected.
- Treatment depends upon the degree of damage to the femoral head. Osteotomy may be required.

Examination tips

- There are five main 'hip X-ray' diagnoses for the examination:
  — Perthes' disease (as demonstrated)
  — slipped upper femoral epiphyses
  — osteomyelitis
  — joint damage due to arthritis
  — developmental dysplasia of the hip.
- Slipped femoral epiphyses should be distinguished by observing the line of the sweep of the femoral neck. Similarly there should not be any evidence of irregularity of the femoral head nor the joint space. The latter may appear superficially narrower because of the posterior displacement of the femoral head.
- The age of detection characteristically differs:
  — Perthes': prepubertal boys
  — slipped epiphyses: peripubertal boys, often overweight, or those children with hypothyroidism.

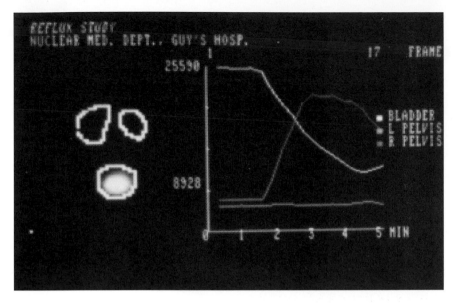

This is a renal DTPA radioisotope scan.

What does it show?

ANSWER 52

This scan shows right reflux.

Comments

- The counts are high in the bladder and then fall during micturition. The counts are lower over the kidneys and they should remain so. However, there is an increase in activity during micturition signifying vesicoureteric reflux.
- This type of scan is dynamic.
- This scan does give an analysis of renal function but it is less accurate than a DMSA scan which is static and also gives a view of the renal structure.

Examination tips

- This sort of information may be encountered in the data interpretation paper as well as part of the investigations in a grey case.

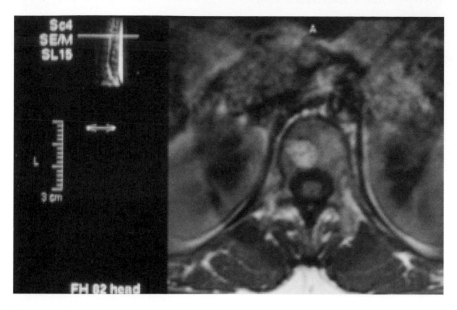

This spinal MRI scan was performed in a teenager with chronic back pain.

a) Describe the abnormality.
b) Give one potential diagnosis.

ANSWER 53

a) Well circumscribed high-signal rounded lesion within the vertebral body.
b) Haemangioma.
  Arteriovenous malformation.
  Vascular malignancy.
  Cyst.

Comments

- As previously mentioned, fluid provides this high signal.
- This appearance is characteristic of haemangioma.
- This was an incidental finding in this patient whose back pain was of psychogenic origin.
- Generally back pain is unusual in children below 12 years and must be taken seriously, particularly as it may be a sign of impending spinal disease such as malignancy.

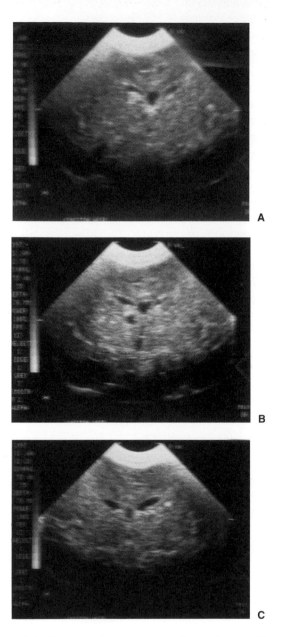

A

B

C

This neonatal cranial ultrasound scan was performed on a 35-week gestation infant who was critically ill with multisystem failure. A profound thrombocytopenia was noted in conjunction with marked hepatosplenomegaly.

a) What abnormalities are noted on the coronal view?
b) What is the most likely diagnosis?
c) How may the diagnosis be confirmed?

ANSWER 54

a) Periventricular calcification.
b) Congenital cytomegalovirus (CMV) infection.
c) Isolation of cytomegalovirus from a urine sample obtained within the first 2 weeks of life.

Comments

- The calcification is best seen in the lower picture as a line of bright dots beneath the ventricle.
- To remember the difference between CMV and toxoplasmosis – CMV usually has periventricular calcification rather than the widespread lesions in toxoplasmosis.
- Many infants with congenital CMV infection are asymptomatic but may develop chorioretinitis later.
- The presence of central nervous system disease is associated with a poorer prognosis.
- Early urinary isolation is important to avoid the possibility that infection is postnatally acquired. Nervous system disease involvement would be rare in this circumstance.
- Serological testing is attractive but CMV-specific IgM titres may be low or even falsely negative in some infants.

Examination tips

- Congenital infections are common questions in the examination.
- CMV infection is still the most common classic congenital infection in the UK.
- Bright echoes on the cranial ultrasound scan may be:
  — calcification
  — haemorrhage
  — infarction or ischaemic changes
  — artefact (particularly the bright parallel lines surrounding the lateral ventricle on the parasagittal view which is an acoustic window – *avoid an incorrect interpretation of germinal matrix haemorrhage*).

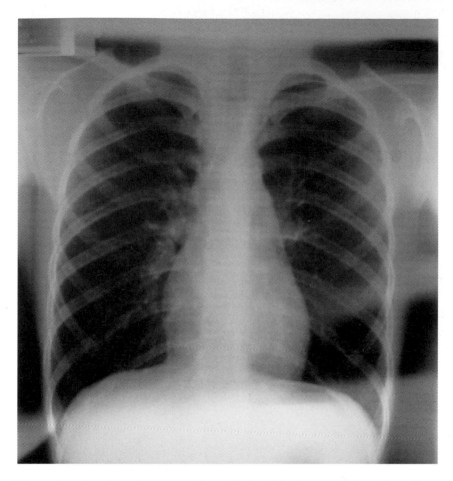

This patient is referred to your chest clinic with the complaint of persistent intermittent cough. A chest X-ray was performed.

a) Describe the abnormality.
b) What is the most likely diagnosis?

ANSWER 55

a) Bilateral hyperinflation.
b) Chronic asthma.

Comments

- Hyperinflation is usually due to air-trapping mechanisms, e.g. asthma, foreign body (if unilateral).
- Hyperinflation is best detected by the overall volume of the lung appearance rather than the traditional anterior rib count plus the flattening of the diaphragm. The heart often appears rather narrow.
- Cough, particularly nocturnal, exercise-induced or laughter-associated, is the most common symptom of asthma.
- The same appearance might be expected in an acute asthma attack with respiratory distress although this is excluded in the examination question introduction.

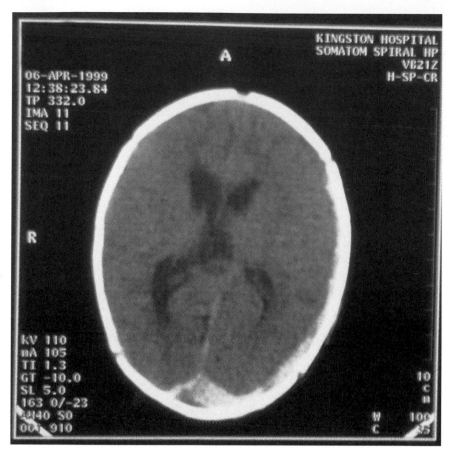

A 5-week-old boy was admitted with a history of apnoeic episodes. He was born at term by a Ventouse delivery. He had received one dose of oral Vitamin K before discharge home. Clinically he appeared pale and his anterior fontanelle was full.

a) What is demonstrated on this scan?
b) Give two possible explanations.

ANSWER 56

a) Bilateral posterior subdural haemorrhage extending forward on the left.
b) Late presenting haemorrhagic disease of the newborn.
   Traumatic subdural haemorrhage (often associated with non-accidental injury).
   Persistent subdural haemorrhage following Ventouse extraction.

Comments

- Subdural haemorrhages are usually narrow haemorrhages which do not bulge into the brain tissue as seen in extradural bleeds.
- They are often anteriorly situated.
- Fresh blood appears white on the scan.
- Ventouse extraction has been recorded as a definite cause of bleeding although the appearance of the bleed now at this age should look hypodense, i.e. blacker.
- Subdural haemorrhages may swell as the blood contained within them is broken down, thereby increasing the osmotic load – this in turn may precipitate further bleeding.
- Subdurals are often associated with child abuse in infants, particularly the shaken baby mechanism whereby the bridging veins are torn as the brain rocks with the movement.
- Intracranial haemorrhage is the most common presentation of late-presenting haemorrhagic disease of the newborn.
- The association of cerebral atrophy with subdural haemorrhage in the absence of a history of trauma or fracture may indicate an underlying metabolic disorder – glutaric aciduria type 1.

Examination tips

- It may be difficult to differentiate between subdural and evidence of atrophy – the history may be of help, as may the appearance of the underlying gyri.
- The dating of subdurals is difficult – a rough guide is as follows: hyperdense blood is within a haemorrhage within the last 36 hours; isodense haemorrhage is within 2–7 days; and hypodense thereafter.
- Often a MRI scan is performed to identify any underlying cerebral damage.

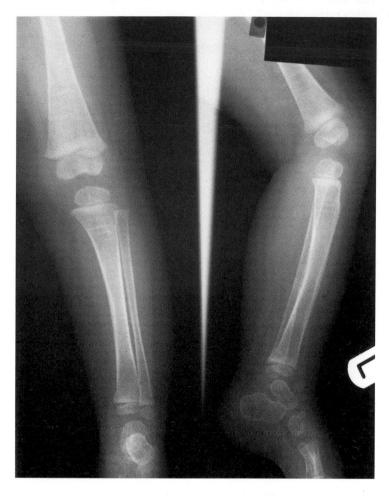

Jemma is an 18-month-old girl undergoing extensive chemotherapy for acute myeloid leukaemia. She presented to the A&E department refusing to weight-bear.

a) Describe two radiological abnormalities.
b) Is this likely to be child abuse?

ANSWER 57

a) Growth arrest lines.
   Metaphyseal buckle fracture.
   Osteopenic bones.
b) No.

Comments

- Note the thin transverse white lines signifying growth arrest – this child had required several cycles of chemotherapy complicated by a coliform septicaemia.
- The small fracture was a buckle stress fracture occurring as a result of the osteopenic bones. This is a common fracture and should not be confused with the bucket handle fractures of the metaphyses seen in child abuse cases.

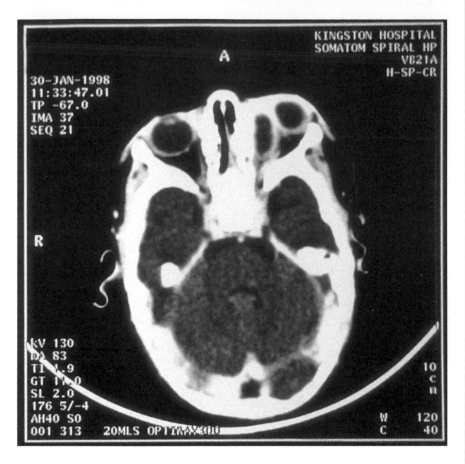

This child was referred by a general practitioner. The child had initially presented the preceding weekend with a history of periorbital erythema which had not settled with oral amoxycillin. The child continued to worsen with a spiking fever of 39.5°C. On admission, there was a neutrophilia and elevated C-reactive protein of 241 mg/L.

a) What is the diagnosis?
b) Which two physical signs should be carefully examined for?
c) Give one potential complication.

ANSWER 58

a) Left retro-orbital abscess with left ethmoid opacity (infection).

b) Proptosis (may be difficult with the degree of soft tissue oedema present). Painful or restricted eye movements.

c) Central nervous system spread including:
- — cavernous sinus thrombosis
- — intracranial abscess
- — meningitis
- — damage to the optic nerve.

Comments

- A fluid level-containing cyst-like structure is identified on the medial wall of the left orbit.
- Taken in conjuction with the history and results, preceding orbital cellulitis has progressed to a retro-orbital abscess.
- The source of the infection may be the sinuses, which should be examined.
- Surgical drainage is often necessary.
- Proptosis and/or painful restricted ocular movements are suggestive that this is not just preseptal periorbital cellulitis. This latter diagnosis is often amenable to oral antibiotic therapy.

Examination tips

- Sites around the sinuses may be difficult. Again, compare sides to ensure that pathology is not missed.
- Retro-orbital masses include:
  - — abscess
  - — tumour (rhabdomyosarcoma)
  - — metastatic disease (neuroblastoma)
  - — malignant extension of (i) osteosarcoma (ii) optic nerve tumour.

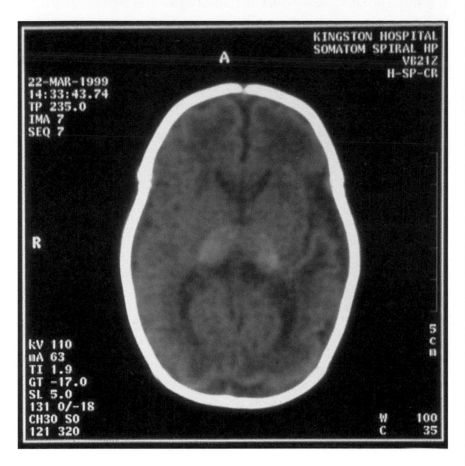

A term infant was born by emergency caesarian section with Apgar scores of 0@1 minute, 2@5 minutes and 6@10 minutes. The cord pH was 6.9 with a base deficit of −20. The infant was intubated and received 40 mL/kg of fluid for resuscitation. A blood glucose level was 1.2 mmol/L. The infant began to suffer generalised seizures from 30 minutes of age, which were controlled with phenobarbitone. A CT scan was performed,

a) What abnormality is demonstrated?
b) What is the prognosis?

ANSWER 59

a) Bilateral thalamic haemorrhage with early signs of cerebral atrophy.
b) Poor.

Comments

- The CT scan shows bright bilateral symmetrical lesions in both thalami. Such appearance usually occurs secondary to ischaemia although it may also be post-haemorrhagic.
- Neurodevelopmental outcome is usually poor as the thalami are major sites of sensory and motor integration.
- Visual defects virtually always occur, often exceeding deficits occurring secondary to occipital cortex damage.
- This is another form of neonatal encephalopathy.

Examination tips

- Try to predict what type of abnormality may be present from the question. The possibilities in this question include:
  — cerebral oedema with ventricular compression
  — poor grey/white matter differentiation
  — subdural haemorrhage
  — cerebral atrophy
  — occasionally cerebral infarct.

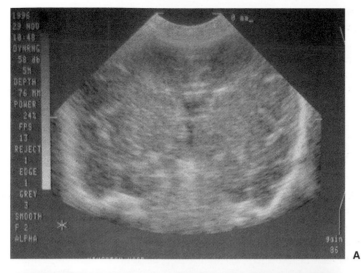

A

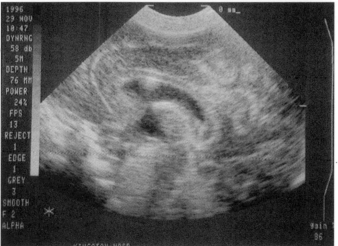

B

Which of the following statements regarding this neonatal cranial ultrasound scan is correct?

a) The scan demonstrates a prominent aqueduct of Sylvius.
b) The scan demonstrates a prominent fourth ventricle.
c) The scan demonstrates a prominent foramen of Munro.
d) The scan demonstrates absence of the septum pellucidum.
e) The scan demonstrates a prominent third ventricle.

ANSWER 60

The correct answer is **(e)**.

Comments

- The slit-like echo-free area in the midline in this coronal section is the third ventricle. It appears as a triangular shape on midline sagittal view.
- This appearance resolves with increasing gestational age.
- The third ventricle connects the lateral ventricles to the aqueduct of Sylvius via the foramen of Munro.
- The curved echo-free area on the sagittal view is the cavum septum pellucidum.

Examination tips

- Try to review as many neonatal cranial ultrasound scans as possible so that pathology and normal variants may be recognised easily.
- The classic examination cases include:
  — intraventricular haemorrhage
  — ventricular dilatation
  — hydrocephalus
  — cysts (see Question 22), including periventricular leucomalacia and porencephaly.

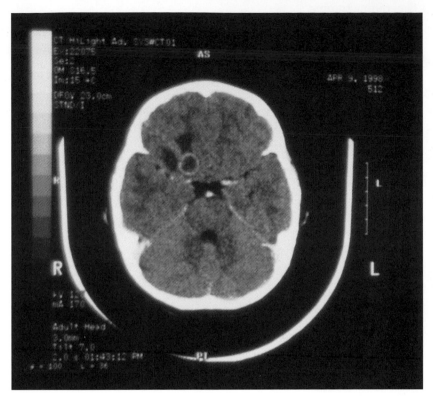

This CT scan was performed on a child with Fallot's tetralogy who developed a fever and drowsiness. This is a contrast study.

a) What is the diagnosis?
b) Give two other possible underlying causes for your diagnosis.

ANSWER 61

a) Right frontal lobe abscess.

b) Penetrating trauma.

ENT infection (otitis media, sinus infection and mastoiditis).

Congenital immunodeficiency.

HIV infection.

Parasitic infection.

Comments

- An enhancing ring shadow is demonstrated which is an abscess. This diagnosis should be considered in those with fever, neurological symptoms/ signs in the presence of cyanotic cardiac disease.
- Abscesses may occur after penetrating trauma and basal skull fractures.
- Direct spread from an ENT infection is a possibility. Spread from the high-pressure environment of an infected sinus down valveless bridging veins into the intracranial cavity may occur.
- Cysticercosis (parasitic infection) is a differential diagnosis in those from risk areas.

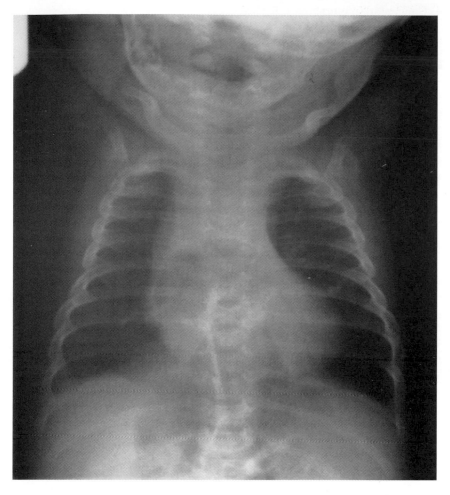

A 4-month-old child was investigated for apnoeic spells. A cranial ultrasound scan, ECG and EEG were normal. A pH probe study indicated a pH index of 30.1%. The chest X-ray is shown.

a) What is demonstrated?
b) Give one differential diagnosis.

ANSWER 62

a) Central hiatus hernia.

b) Congenital diaphragmatic hernia.
   Achalasia.

Comments

- A dark shadow may be discerned through the mediastinal shadow. This has the typical shape of an abdominal hernia. This hernia has exacerbated the underlying reflux as shown by the severely abnormal pH probe study.
- Late presentations of congenital diaphragmatic herniae have been reported, although a neonatal presentation with hypoxia and respiratory failure is more commonplace.
- Traumatic herniae can occur.
- Herniation due to congenital diaphragmatic hernia is most commonly left-sided.
- Achalasia is rare in infants.

Examination tips

- Always try to look through the mediastinal shadow to exclude hidden pathology. This is particularly important to exclude left basal pneumonia.
- Always trace the path of both hemidiaphragms to exclude hidden basal pathology.
- Occasionally a lateral view will be given and may be invaluable.

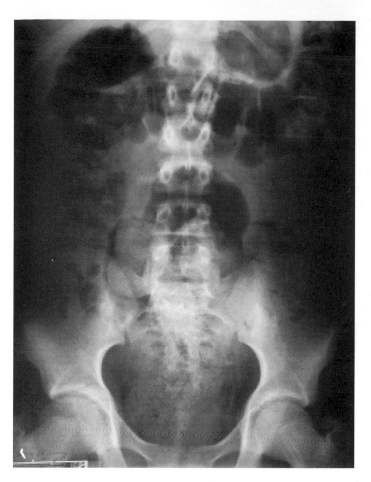

A 7-year-old boy presented to the A&E department with severe abdominal colic. This X-ray was arranged.

What is the most likely diagnosis?

ANSWER 63

Marked faecal loading indicating constipation.

Comments

- Constipation is usually diagnosed clinically without resort to radiology. However, such a film may be invaluable when parental acceptance of the diagnosis is in doubt.
- The lower colon and rectum may contain rounded faecal residue. More proximal bowel shows a speckled pattern of faeces. Gaseous distension may be seen. This may be severe and outline the haustrae particularly of the transverse colon.
- Constipation may be a feature of:
  — neuropathic rectum
  — hypothyroidism
  — Hirschsprung's disease
  — post-GI surgery
  — cow's milk protein intolerance
  — hypercalcaemia
  — feeding problems with inadequate fluid intake
  — syndromes, e.g. Down syndrome
  — behavioural/emotional problems often in association with stool holding or encopresis.

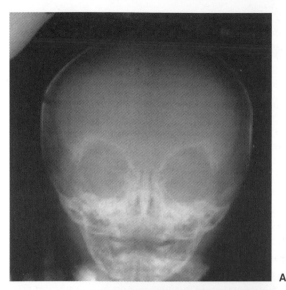

A

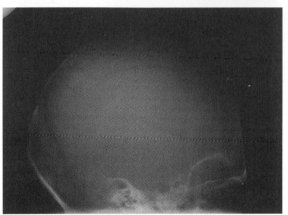

B

A 5-week-old girl was admitted having been accidentally knocked out of her car seat by her sibling aged 4 years. She had not been strapped in at the time.

a) What abnormalities are shown?
b) What other steps would you now take and why?

127

ANSWER 64

a) Bilateral wide skull fractures extending anteriorly along the whole length of the parietal bones.

b) (i) Urgent CT brain scan to ensure that there is no underlying intracranial injury.

(ii) Consider a child protection investigation – the force required to produce such fractures is not compatible with the history of a trivial fall. The bilateral nature of the fractures suggests that an alternative story of injury is likely.

Comments

- The following are the standard quoted features of skull fractures likely to be of a non-accidental nature:
  — multiple
  — branched
  — wide
  — occipital – the thickness of this bone usually precludes trivial injury as a cause
  — bilateral parietal
  — affecting more than one bone
  — multiple depressed
  — associated with intracranial injury.
- In the absence of other features, osteogenesis imperfecta is a very rare cause of skull fracture.
- Always arrange a fundoscopic examination for retinal haemorrhages.
- A skeletal survey should be performed.

Examination tips

- Rehearse the steps required in the evaluation of a case of suspected child abuse as this is a popular examination topic, particularly in the oral section.

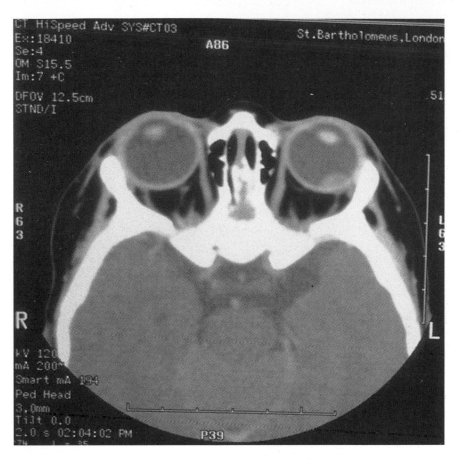

This baby was referred for assessment of a squint. An abnormality was noted which precipitated the performing of this investigation.

a) What abnormality is likely to have been noted?
b) What is the diagnosis?
c) What long-term complication is possible?

ANSWER 65

a) Left leucocoria.
b) Left retinoblastoma.
c) Late-presenting secondary tumours.

Comments

- Quoted incidence of 1:18 000 live births.
- 60% are sporadic but 40% are familial.
- A two-stage hit mutation hypothesis of the Rb1 gene is envisaged. Both retinal or germ cells can be affected – the latter will cause bilateral disease.
- Leucocoria occurs in 60%.
  — management is variable but may include:
  — chemotherapy
  — radiotherapy – external and local
  — cryotherapy
  — surgical enucleation.
- This CT confirms a retinal mass without retro orbital extension.

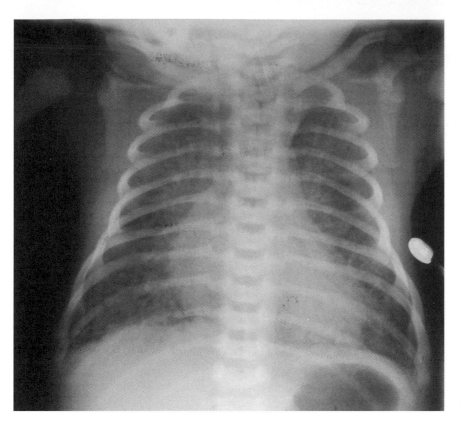

A baby is admitted to the neonatal unit on the day of discharge because of mild cyanosis. No abnormality had been noted on the initial day 1 neonatal examination. Now, on day 5, the baby had a short ejection systolic murmur with an ECG suggesting borderline biventricular hypertrophy.

What is the most likely diagnosis?

ANSWER 66

Transposition of the great arteries with a ventricular septal defect (VSD).

Comments

- 20% of infants with a transposition also have a VSD. This alters their clinical presentation.
- Unlike uncomplicated transposition, these infants rarely manifest their cardiac status within the first 24 hours.
- Cyanosis is usually mild. Cardiomegaly occurs and failure ensues if the diagnosis is missed.
- Pulmonary plethora may occur, as in this case.
- The narrow vasculature pedicle occurs.
- Treatment is usually with emergency septostomy followed by an arterial switch procedure thereafter.

Examination tips

- It is often difficult to make a firm diagnosis on chest X-ray alone.
- *A useful approach is:*
  - cardiac size (check type of view and degree of rotation and inspiration)
  - cardiac shape (beware the large thymus)
  - plethora or oligaemic lungfields?
  - hepatic shadow enlarged?
  - pulmonary oedema?
  - signs of previous cardiac surgery – clips or sternal sutures.
- *Some classics include:*
  - narrow pedicle with plethoric or normal lungs = transposition
  - large heart with plethora = hypoplastic left heart syndrome
  - normal heart with oligaemia = Fallot's tetralogy
  - boot-shaped heart with oligaemia = pulmonary atresia with VSD
  - square-shaped heart with oligaemia = tricuspid atresia.

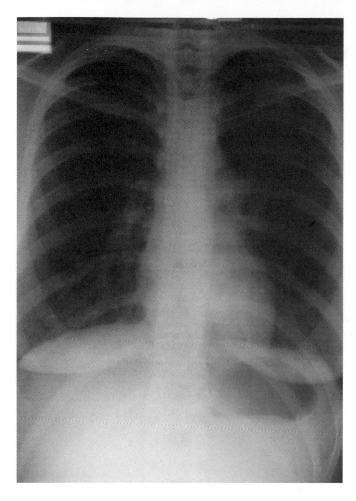

This child was referred following pre-BCG school screening. She was asymptomatic.

a) Describe the abnormality.
b) What is your management?
c) The school wishes to know whether they need to undertake any special precautions. What is your answer?

ANSWER 67

a) Pulmonary tuberculosis with left regional lymphadenopathy (Ghon complex) with calcification.

b) Contact tracing to identify the index case.
Full chemotherapy.

c) Unlikely, as few children are smear-positive and are therefore rarely infectious.

Comments

- Cavitating disease is rare in children.
- Primary TB is often asymptomatic and only detected by an abnormal tuberculin test and abnormal chest X-ray.
- CT scans may identify hilar lymphadenopathy not readily seen on chest X-ray.
- Abnormal radiological features include:
  — lymph node calcification
  — upper lobe streaking
  — peripheral calcification
  — mediastinal lymphadenopathy
  — persistent collapse due to endobronchial node disease.
- It is rare to obtain an organism by bronchoscopy.

Examination tips

- It is easy to over-interpret hilar lymphadenopathy – it will be severe if presented in the examination.
- Know the national guidelines.

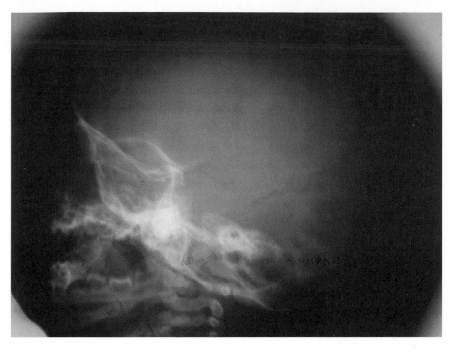

What normal variant is shown on this X-ray?

ANSWER 68

Wormian bone.

Comments
- Wormian bones are islands of skull surrounded by sutures.
- They may be normal variants.
- They are seen frequently in those with skeletal disease, particularly relatives of those with brittle bone diseases.

Examination tips
- Do not mistake these suture extensions as fracture lines. Suture lines are generally much more erratic and very thin.

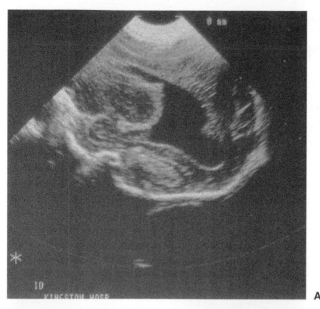

A

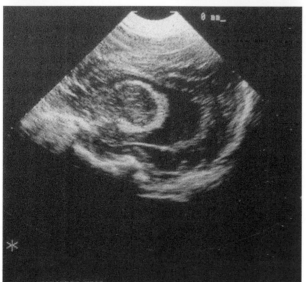

B

This is a neonatal cranial ultrasound scan of a preterm infant of 27 weeks' gestation who is now 28 days of age.

What is shown?

ANSWER 69

Lateral ventricle dilatation.

Comments

- This parasagittal view shows that the ventricle is dilated rather than the slit-like curved appearance normally seen.
- This may occur with or without preceding bleeding.
- Usually the dilatation spontaneously arrests and does not progress onto hydrocephalus.
- Serial scans are often needed with the measurement of ventricular index.
- Ventricular index is the maximal width of the lateral ventricle in the coronal plane measured from the midline.

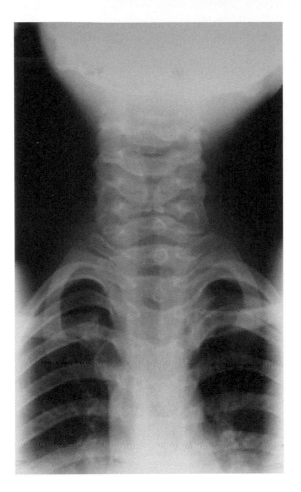

A 5-year-old boy was referred following his fourth admission with stridor which was believed to be due to viral croup. Further investigations were performed.

a) What is shown?
b) Give one further investigation to aid diagnosis.

ANSWER 70

a) Minor subglottic narrowing.
b) Direct laryngobronchoscopy.

Comments

- Straight X-rays of the neck are difficult to interpret. Some authorities suggest a Cincinnati view which is a high-voltage filtered view of the subglottic airway. However, even this film gives a suggestion of a narrowing.
- Direct visual inspection is often necessary.
- A structural predisposing lesion is suggested by virtue of the frequent history of croup in an older child.
- Other lesions, such as a double aortic arch, may need exclusion, although presentation is usually at a younger age. This may be suggested by barium studies and confirmed by MRI.

Examination tips

- Other 'neck' diagnoses include:
  — foreign body
  — retropharyngeal oedema/abscess
  — curled feeding tubes in oesophageal atresia
  — skeletal abnormalities such as erosion of vertebrae or fractures
  — hyoid bone fracture
  — calcified cervical lymph nodes.
- As with other X-rays, do not miss other pathology. Have a system such as:
  — look for tubes etc.
  — check the airway
  — check the prevertebral space
  — check the appearance of the vertebrae
  — check the hyoid bone
  — check the extracervical soft tissue, e.g. nodes
  — check the clavicles (fracture?).

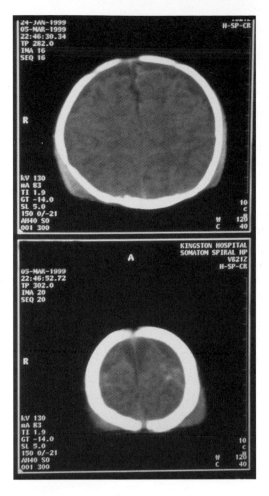

This CT scan was performed on a small child who had been involved in a serious car accident. The plain skull X-ray confirmed a fracture.

What does this film show?

ANSWER 71

Evidence of fresh bleeding in left side of brain – this was a subarachnoid haemorrhage.

There is also evidence of an older subdural haemorrhage on the same side.

Comments

- As previously mentioned, bright substances on CT often represent fresh bleeding. It is difficult to be sure whether this is intracerebral or subarachnoid in origin. A darker old subdural was present (the darker crescent in the left anterior area) and the cause of this was uncertain.
- Subarachnoid bleeding may be spontaneous or associated with trauma.
- As already discussed, subdurals in infants are usually due to shearing forces such as that encountered in shaking episodes.
- Note the extracranial soft tissue swelling bilaterally.

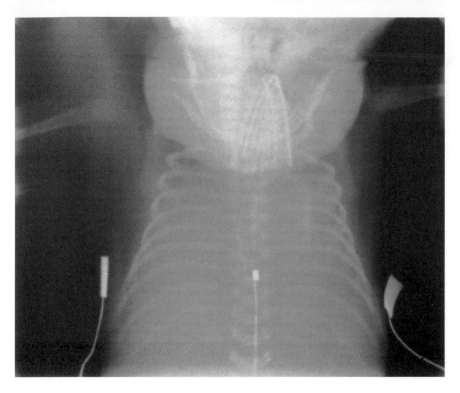

This X-ray belongs to an infant of 846 g, born at 27 weeks' gestation, who was admitted to the neonatal unit. The arterial blood gases showed: pH 7.24, P_{CO_2} = 6.4 kPa, P_{O_2} = 4.6 kPa, HCO_3 = 16.4 mmol/L, BXs = –5.4.

a) Give two major differential diagnoses.
b) What is your next line of action?

ANSWER 72

a) Surfactant deficient hyaline membrane disease (respiratory distress syndrome).
   Group B beta-haemolytic streptococcal sepsis.
b) Improved ventilatory support with the instillation of exogenous surfactant.

Comments

- There is widespread bilateral shadowing of the lungs.
- Mediastinal definition is difficult as a result of severe lung disease.
- The lungs are of low volume – suggestive of surfactant deficiency.
- Such babies are also treated for sepsis with antibiotics.
- Exogenous surfactant has altered the natural history of respiratory distress syndrome.
- Sepsis may present with refractory hypoxia with reasonable CO_2 excretion which suggests pulmonary hypertension; this may be treated with vasodilators or, more recently, inhaled nitric oxide.

Examination tips

- Check the size of the lung fields to see whether this may be surfactant deficiency.
- The size of lung fields is also important in meconium aspiration and during oscillatory ventilation.
- Note the position of the endotracheal tube (rather high) and that of the nasogastric tube and umbilical arterial catheter.

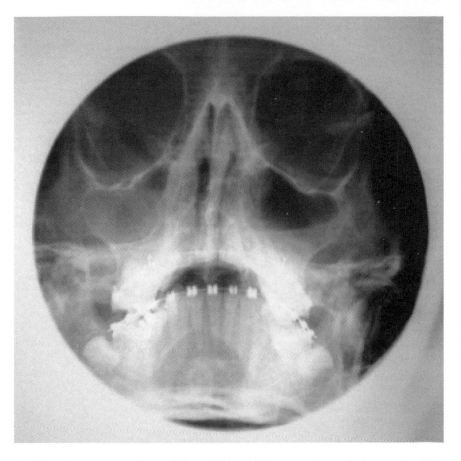

A plain X-ray was performed in a child with fever and nasal obstruction. The child had a long history of chronic cough.

What is demonstrated?

ANSWER 73

Bilateral maxillary sinusitis.

Comments

- Note the fluid levels – the most reliable radiological sign of sinusitis.
- The maxillary sinuses and ethmoidal sinuses are most frequently involved as they develop at an earlier age.
- Maxillary sinuses may cause facial and oral pain.
- The causative organisms may be mixed respiratory flora.

Examination tips

- Features also suggestive of sinus disease include:
  - — opacity of sinus
  - — haziness of sinus
  - — haziness with indistinct borders.
- Check other sinuses to see whether they are involved, such as the paranasal ethmoid sinuses and the frontal sinuses, but bear in mind the age of sinus development.

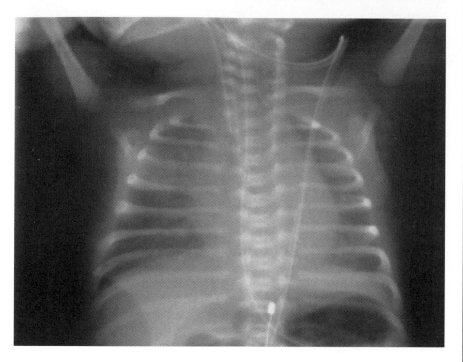

You are asked to review this neonatal chest X-ray following a procedure.

a) What abnormality is unearthed on inspection?
b) What precaution may occasionally be needed?

ANSWER 74

a) Abnormally sited percutaneous Silastic long line – inserted via a left antecubital fossa vein but diverting up the left internal jugular vein.
b) The site of the line must always be verified before use. This may sometimes necessitate the introduction of a radio-opaque medium to identify the tip of the line.

Comments

- As previously mentioned, it is good practice to check for the position of any central/long line prior to its use.
- Complications of neonatal long lines include:
  — infection
  — migration into other vascular areas
  — rupture of vein leading to TPN accumulation, e.g. in lung
  — thrombosis
  — mechanical problems.
- Note the increased shadowing of the right upper lobe and the endotracheal tube.

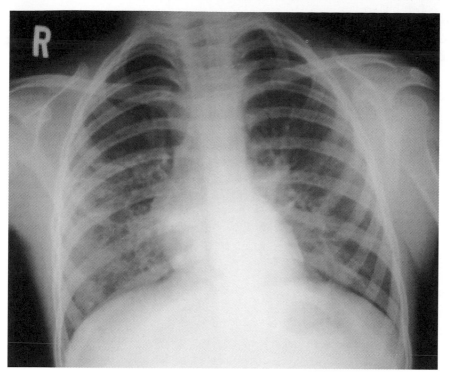

This 8-year-old girl was rescued from a house fire. She was given oxygen in the ambulance. This is her X-ray.

a) Describe two abnormalities.
b) What is the likely diagnosis?
c) Give one further useful investigation.

ANSWER 75

a) Diffuse bilateral lower lobe reticular shadowing.
   Left hilar collapse.
b) Smoke inhalation with subsequent pneumonitis.
c) Arterial blood gas.
   Carboxyhaemoglobin estimation.

Comments

- Damage to the airway may be due to the toxic effects of heat, smoke particles, toxic gas and the secondary effects, e.g. hypoxia.
- The end result is a combination of pneumonitis, pulmonary oedema, secondary pneumonia, atelectasis and carbon monoxide poisoning.
- Prompt treatment to avoid these issues is of paramount importance.
- This child required hyperbaric oxygen therapy to aid correction of her carbon monoxide poisoning. Most authorities agree that a carboxy-haemoglobin estimate > 40% is an indication for this therapy.
- Stridor due to upper airway damage may coexist.

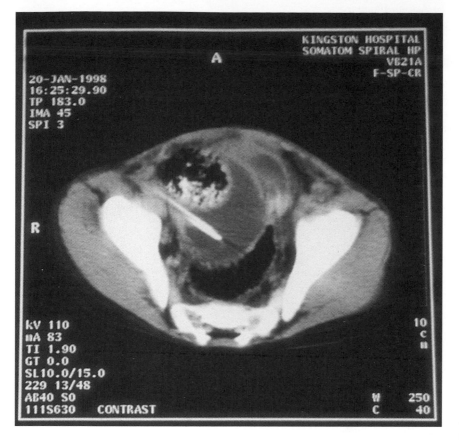

A 10-year-old child was admitted with a history of central abdominal pain. Her white count was elevated as was her C-reactive protein (CRP) at 75 mg/L. Her pain localised to the right iliac fossa but then subsided. She continued to spike a fever above 39.5°C. Her abdomen was generally tender without bowel sounds. Her CRP rose over 24 hours to 251 mg/L. After an abdominal ultrasound scan, this investigation was organised.

a) What is demonstrated?
b) What is the most likely diagnosis?

ANSWER 76

a) Fluid-filled mass in the abdominal cavity containing a surgical drain.
b) Appendix abscess.

Comments

- The history is suggestive of appendicitis. Upon appendiceal rupture, the acute pain may subside with either the production of a walled abscess or spread to cause peritonitis.
- The differential diagnosis would also include Crohn's disease. A psoas abscess is retroperitoneal.
- Ultrasound scans may be useful in the diagnosis of appendicitis in experienced hands where a prominent appendix shadow may be identified due to oedema.
- Despite apparent clinical amelioration, the blood investigations signify worsening inflammation/infection.
- Note the low-density centre of the mass, indicating fluid.

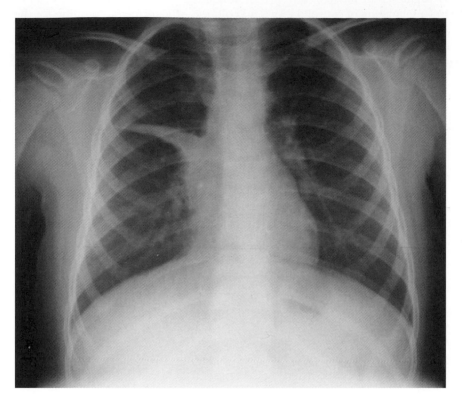

This is a child with a fever.

a) Anatomically where does the pathology lie?
b) What is the most likely cause of this appearance?
c) In what circumstances would you advise a further chest X-ray?

ANSWER 77

a) Right middle lobe.

b) Combination of consolidation and collapse – the former accounting for the fever and the latter because there is suggestion of some slight volume loss in the right upper lobe.

c) *Acutely*: if there is clinical deterioration or the clinical signs alter to suggest an effusion.

Chronically: the indications for a follow-up X-ray are debated but most clinicians would include:

- lobar pneumonia – to ensure resolution, i.e. that there is no segmental obstruction
- coexisting effusion
- right middle lobe changes – these can be difficult to clear without prolonged physiotherapy
- persisting symptoms or signs
- where the underlying diagnosis is endobronchial tuberculosis
- after pertussis or measles – to exclude early bronchiectasis
- in cystic fibrosis
- after a foreign body – some authorities suggest the use of ventilation/ perfusion scans to ensure complete resolution after lung involvement with a foreign body.

Comments

- The X-ray outlines a clear linear shadow sitting on the horizontal fissure.
- Remember that the right lung has three lobes, whereas the left has two lobes with the upper including the lingular segment.
- Significant right upper lobe collapse may manifest radiologically with volume loss as shown by the raising of the horizontal fissure. Other lobes may be affected but are harder to identify as they may be masked by compensatory hyperinflation of the adjacent lobe.
- Pneumonia may be shown as:
  — lobar
  — bronchopneumonic
  — round
  — loss of the hemidiaphragm shadow
  — cavitating lesion appearing as an abscess
  — perimediastinal shadow
  — loss of the definition of the heart border (right middle lobe or left lingular).

Examination tips

- Check for associated radiological signs to confirm your diagnosis or clinical suspicion.
- Check the question for any suggestion of:
  — cystic fibrosis
  — aspiration
  — immunodeficiency
  — tuberculosis.

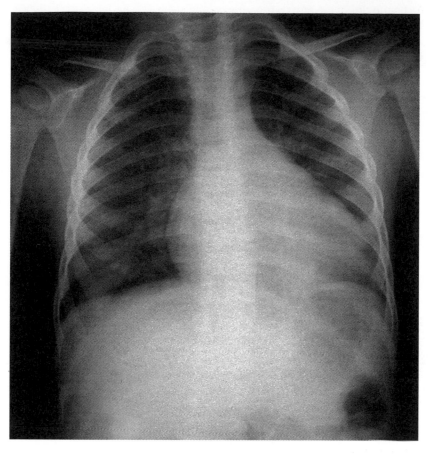

A 4-year-old African boy was admitted with breathlessness and a non-productive cough. His haemoglobin was 5.3 g/dL. He had previously been admitted with a febrile illness associated with swelling of his fingers. His CRP was 36 mg/L. His blood film was hypochromic and microcytic.

a) What is the most likely underlying diagnosis?
b) Give one test to confirm your diagnosis.
c) What does this X-ray show?

ANSWER 78

a) Sickle cell disease.
b) Haemoglobin electrophoresis.
c) Left ventricular enlargement (presumed hypertrophy).

Comments

- Cardiac abnormalities are quite common in children with sickle disease even if they have not been overtransfused.
- An echocardiogram will give more useful information.
- Lobar changes in sickle cell disease may indicate:
  — sickle chest syndrome (combination of sequestration, infarction and infection)
  — pneumonia.
- This child's initial presentation was dactylitis.
- If this child did not have sickle disease, then the features may be compatible with an early cardiomyopathy.

Examination tips

- The main sickle crises include:
  — painful/vaso-occlusive
  — aplastic (due to parvovirus infection)
  — infective
  — sequestrative (usually abdominal affecting the spleen in infants)
  — neurological (with stroke)
  — megaloblastic.
- Sickle disease is popular, particularly examining knowledge of presentations such as dactylitis.
- Sickle cell blood films are possible photographic cases.

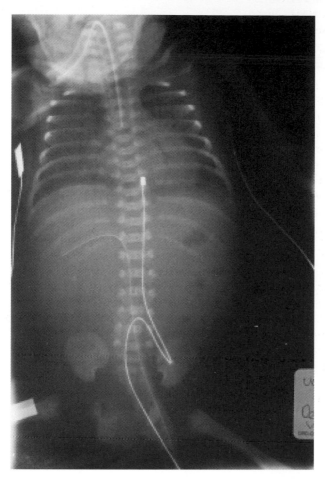

List the iatrogenic added shadows seen on this X-ray of a preterm infant.

ANSWER 79

Umbilical arterial line.
Umbilical venous line.
Endotracheal tube.
Surface electrodes.

Comments

- *Umbilical arterial line* – these dip down before joining the aorta and proceeding up in the midline. Units differ in their choice of preferred location of the tip of the line. Some prefer lower lines sitting at approximately L4. These may be associated with a shorter life and possibly vascular complications. Others prefer higher lines at the level of the diaphragm, although concerns exist about the effect on the mesenteric blood flow. *Always* avoid the position of the renal arteries at L1 level.
- *Umbilical venous line* – this does not dip down but its path upwards is not in the midline. Often the line will deviate into liver or else pass through the ductus venosus and enter the right atrium.
- *Endotracheal tube* – ensure that this does not enter the right main bronchus (see Question 6) nor sit abutting the carina where respiratory movements may impede delivery of oxygen or result in misplacement into the right main bronchus.

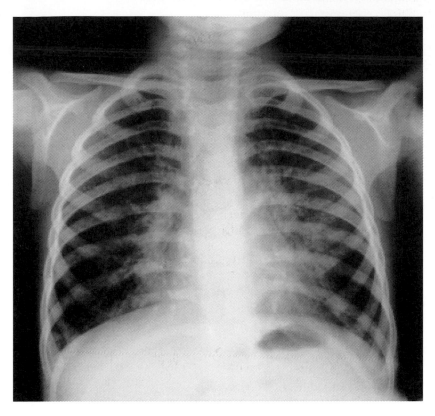

A 10-year-old child was seen with a respiratory infection with marked cough. She presented with a widespread rounded erythematous rash and arthralgia. Her fingers felt very cold but her pulses were normal. Her capillary refill time was 2 seconds. Her CRP was 67 mg/L. Her ESR was 79 mm/hour. Blood film confirmed rouleaux formation. Her blood cultures were negative.

a) Describe the radiological abnormality.
b) What is the most likely causative organism?
c) From the history, what is the rash?

ANSWER 80

a) Bilateral lower and middle lobe bronchopneumonia.
b) *Mycoplasma pneumoniae* infection.
c) Erythema multiforme.

Comments

- The X-ray confirms widespread bronchopneumonia;the history suggests a multisystem infection; the rash and arthralgia are in keeping with a *Mycoplasma* infection.
- The X-ray changes may seem more marked than clinical examination would suggest.
- Diagnosis is supported by the rouleaux production – the cold peripheries were due to cold agglutinins which are supportive but not diagnostic of the infection.
- Diagnosis was by paired serological titres.
- *Mycoplasma* infection may be responsible for a host of clinical features, which include (not exhaustive list):
  — encephalitis
  — transverse myelitis
  — Guillain–Barré type illness
  — thrombocytopenia
  — haemolytic anaemia
  — pancreatitis
  — hepatitis
  — erythema multiforme
  — bullous myringitis.

Examination tips

- When confronted with a myriad clinical features in association with an infection, consider *Mycoplasma* as a cause; previously it was syphilis in adult medicine.
- Also consider systemic lupus erythematosus (SLE).

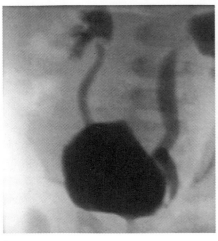

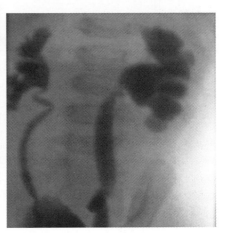

A   B

a) What is the diagnosis?
b) In a young boy, what possible other underlying diagnosis must be considered?

ANSWER 81

a) Bilateral marked (grade IV) vesicoureteric reflux.
b) Posterior urethral valves

Comments

- The management of bilateral antenatal renal dilatation remains controversial. Most authorities suggest early ultrasound scanning, antibiotic prophylaxis and early MCUG to exclude the risk of posterior urethral valve disease.
- Posterior urethral valves are unlikely in this case as the bladder is not enlarged.
- Mothers should always be questioned about their male baby's urinary stream at presentation.

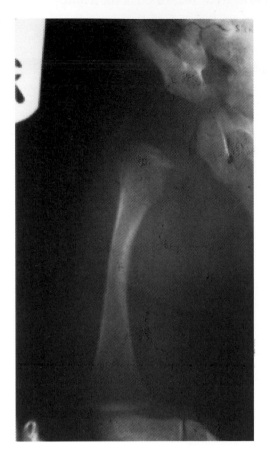

This child refuses to walk or weight-bear. Mother noted a swelling over the upper leg since picking the child up from a childminder.

What can be determined?

ANSWER 82

Spiral fracture through the lower third of the femur.

Comments

- Some films may be difficult to interpret and spiral fractures may be missed!
- The specificity of a long bone fracture for child abuse is at best questionable. A spiral fracture does indicate a twisting force but this does not necessarily mean child abuse.
- A spiral fracture in an active toddler with a good history of injury which has been witnessed is unlikely to be non-accidental in origin.
- No action was necessary from an orthopaedic perspective.

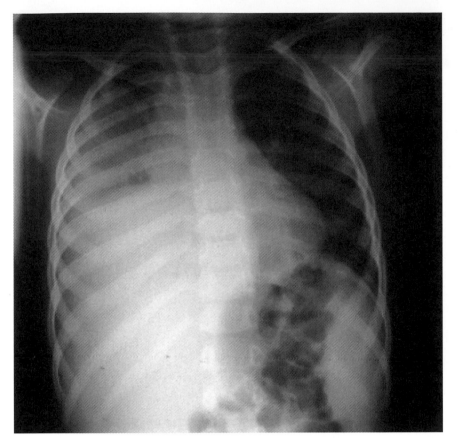

The above chest X-ray was obtained in a 5-year-old girl with breathlessness and high fever. Her temperature failed to settle with antibiotics. Her respiratory examination revealed reduced breath sounds on the right side.

What is the most likely diagnosis?

ANSWER 83

Severe right pleural effusion or empyema.

Comments

- The X-ray suggests that there is an almost complete white shadow affecting the left side with some air visible just at the apex. Taking into account the history, this is most likely an effusion or an empyema.
- This should be ultrasounded to see whether loculation had occurred and to aid diagnostic thoracentesis.
- Always consider malignancy and tuberculosis – obtain a pleural biopsy if possible.

Examination tips

- The typical meniscus appearance may be absent if the volume of pleural fluid is large or if the patient is investigated while supine, when the outline of the lung may be visible as seen in Question 7.
- Most authorities now advocate early pleural aspiration to determine ongoing management, i.e. distinguish between a pleural effusion and an empyema.

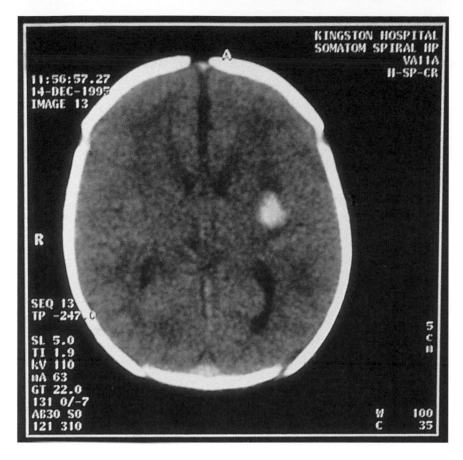

This neonate suffered perinatal asphyxia but has persistent seizures despite appropriate anticonvulsant therapy. This CT scan was obtained.

a) Describe the abnormality shown.
b) Where anatomically is this lesion?
c) Give two differential diagnoses.

ANSWER 84

a) Bright unilateral left echodensity.
b) Left basal ganglia.
c) Calcification following old bleed or ischaemia.
   Fresh local haemorrhage (unlikely due to the history).

Comments

- Another case of neonatal encephalopathy.
- This was calcification.
- Other causes of calcification on a CT scan include:
  — tumour
  — congenital CMV infection
  — other congenital infections – mainly toxoplasmosis
  — infarction
  — pineal gland
  — parasitic cyst
  — metastatic calcification
  — tuberous sclerosis
  — Sturge–Weber syndrome (best seen as tramline calcification on the cerebral surface on plain X-ray).

A boy was referred by the surgical team from the clinic where he was undergoing follow-up following a head injury 9 months previously. On that occasion he had received a high-impact frontal head injury falling off his bicycle. His Glasgow Coma Score at worst was 9/15. His acute CT scans suggested frontal contusion. Since then he has been excessively moody and difficult to control according to his parents. He only complains of mild headaches. Therefore a CT scan was arranged.

a) Give two differential diagnoses.
b) Is the answer to (a) related to his head injury.

ANSWER 85

a) Area of low density in the right frontal lobe. The possible differential include:
— focal atrophy
— arachnoid cyst.

b) Possibly, but not proven!

Comments

- The history and findings are strongly suggestive of focal atrophy following substantial but limited damage to the frontal cortex.
- An arachnoid cyst is usually more basal and lies in the region of the fourth ventricle although there is no reason for it not to occur here. It arises as an indrawing of the arachnoid membrane following inflammatory or traumatic lesions.

Examination tips

- Distinguish this from the appearance of a chronic subdural haematoma. The latter is usually a thin crescent-like lesion, as shown in other preceding cases.

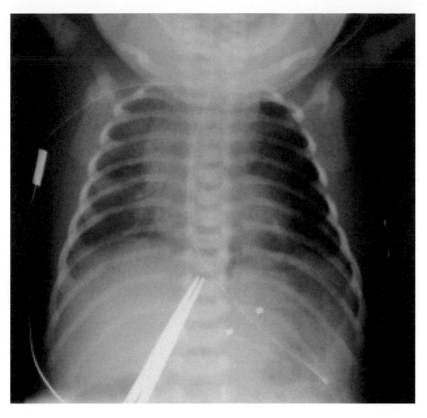

This chest X-ray was performed on an infant whose antenatal period had been complicated by fetal pleural effusions.

a) Describe the chest X-ray.
b) What is the probable explanation for this?

ANSWER 86

a) Radio opaque foreign bodies – apparently in the abdomen.
b) This is a foreign body – in this case an in utero chest drain with metallic markers. The upper marker is actually on the surface of the skin whilst the lower marker is in the lower pleural space (and not the abdominal cavity!).

Comments

- Note that objects low down in the posterior pleural space may appear intra abdominal to the unwary.
- With advances in fetal medicine, fetal surgical techniques are being perfected. The neonatal paediatrician may encounter infants who have undergone the introduction of chest drains or nephrostomies or even cardiac surgery.
- Always check the back of all newborn infants!

Examination tips

- Although candidates wil not be examined on fetal medicine, a basic knowledge is expected at the level that a practising paediatrician is understood to know. Therefore, be aware of the practicalities and the possible therapeutic interventions.
- Know some of the standard presenting problems and their differential diagnoses, e.g. fetal ascites; fetal pleural effusions.
- Rehearse the subsequent neonatal management of antenatally diagnosed problems, e.g. hydronephrosis.

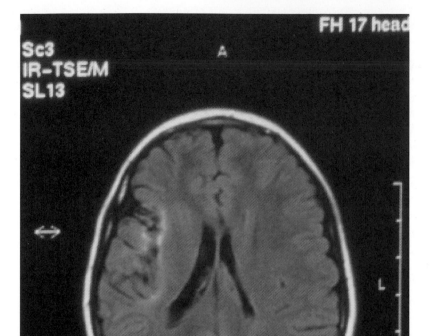

This MRI scan was performed on a child whose head circumference had fallen to below the third centile. The child was born at term to a mother who admitted polydrug abuse which included crack cocaine. The child had suffered two afebrile seizures during the first 3 days associated with hyponatraemia.

a) What is demonstrated?
b) What is the most likely cause?

ANSWER 87

a) Cerebral atrophy around the right Sylvian fissure.

b) The cerebral atrophy may be a result of:
— antenatal problems such as cerebral infarction possibly due to maternal cocaine use
— atrophy secondary to the seizures which themselves may have been due to either drug withdrawal or hyponatraemia.

Comments

- Note cerebral asymmetry.
- Maternal cocaine use may result in fetal cerebral infarction due to its vasoconstrictive effect. This may result in cerebral atrophy.
- Seizures may occur as part of opiate withdrawal.
- Hyponatraemia may occur due to the effects of drug withdrawal on vasopressin release.
- The effects of withdrawal are increasingly difficult to predict in cases where multiple drugs have been used.
- It is difficult to predict the clinical effects of any degree of cerebral atrophy which has a spectrum from severe neurological impairment to outwardly normal development and behaviour.

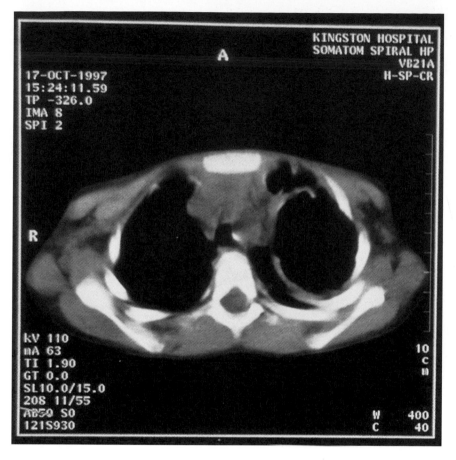

What is the correct interpretation of this thoracic CT scan?

ANSWER 88

Left upper lobe congenital lung cyst.

Comments

- Note the thin-walled structure with absent lung tissue. The thickness of this makes an abscess or pneumatocele unlikely.
- Compare with the plain X-ray appearance in Question 15.

Examination tips

- Other potential CT thorax pathologies include:
  — cystic adenomatoid malformation
  — sequestered lobe
  — bronchiectasis
  — tuberculous lymph node
  — metastatic deposit
  — non-lung pathology, e.g. posterior mediastinal neuroblastoma.

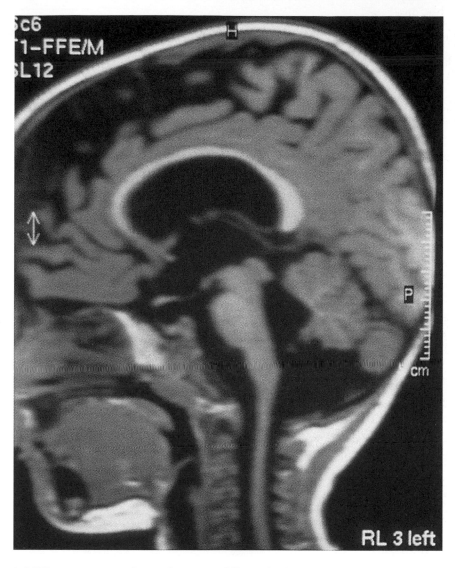

Sc6
T1-FFE/M
SL12

H

P

cm

RL 3 left

A MRI scan was performed on a toddler who had slowed in attaining his motor skills. His head circumference was accelerating through to above the 97th centile. His birth history was unremarkable.

a) What does this scan demonstrate?
b) List three potential underlying diagnoses.

ANSWER 89

a) Sagittal scan showing communicating hydrocephalus.
b) Congenital.
   Idiopathic.
   Associated with syndrome.
   Associated with intracranial infection.
   Associated with intracranial haemorrhage.
   Associated with spinal anomaly.

Comments

- All the intracerebral fluid spaces are dilated suggesting that this is communicating.
- The problem is therefore either cerebral atrophy (unlikely as the head circumference is increasing rapidly) or else a block to CSF circulation elsewhere. This may be a result of an undiagnosed problem with the arachnoid granulation apparatus or a CSF block in the lower spine.
- This case was idiopathic.
- In other cases, consider the above causes plus obstructive tumours and aqueductal stenosis, which may be syndromic (abnormal adducted thumb position) or non-syndromic.
- There may also be evidence of cerebral atrophy.

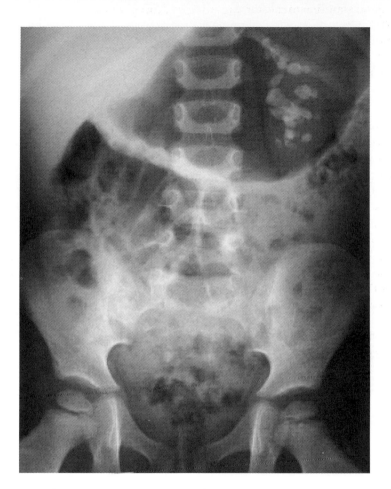

A boy was referred with the diagnosis of a *Proteus* urinary tract infection. This had been associated with haematuria, loin pain, fever and vomiting.

a) What is the diagnosis?
b) Give one further useful investigation to aid further management.
c) What is the most likely outcome?

ANSWER 90

a) Left staghorn renal calculus.
b) DMSA isotope scan to determine degree of residual renal function.
c) Nephrectomy.

Comments

- The radio-opaque calculi branching into the calyceal system can be seen through the dilated stomach gas bubble.
- This is probably a quaternary ammonium salt calculus associated with the urease-producing *Proteus* infection.
- The calculus is too large for lithotripsy.
- The surrounding kidney was severely damaged.

Examination tips

- Try to predict what you may see – the question strongly hints that a calculus will be present (the haematuria, probable pyelonephritis and the causative organism).
- Look in the corners of the X-ray field and the corners of the X-ray film as previously discussed.

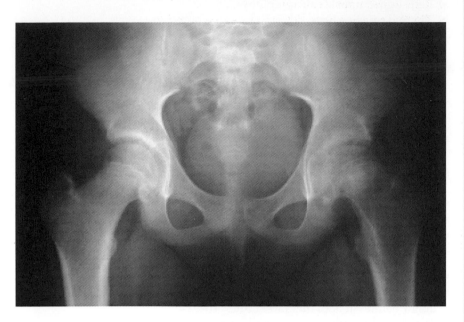

This X-ray belongs to a 10-year-old boy who was referred with a mildly painful limp. He localised the pain to the front of his left thigh. His weight is above the 90th centile and his height is on the 10th centile.

a) What is the diagnosis ?
b) Give one further investigation which may be of help in his management.

ANSWER 91

a) Left slipped upper femoral epiphysis.
b) Thyroid function tests.

Comments

- The film shows an abnormality of the femoral head arrangement. This is identified by tracing the neck of the femur and the femoral head. In comparison to the unaffected side, the orientation of the head has 'slipped' backwards. Although this tends to render the joint space less conspicuous, there is no evidence of erosive joint disease.
- The normal rounded femoral head is preserved, thus helping to exclude Perthes' disease.
- This problem tends to cause a moderately painful limp, but maximal tenderness is usually localised to the thigh or knee.
- There is an increased incidence in peripubertal children where there may be an imbalance between growth factors and steroids.
- It is also seen in acquired hypothyroidism.
- Treatment is surgical with fixation of the femoral head.

Examination tips

- Be sure of the different presentations, clinical features and radiological abnormalities in both this and Perthes' disease.
- Have a regular scheme for looking at hip X-rays, such as:
  — regularity of femoral head
  — position of femoral head
  — appearance of joint space
  — degree of mineralisation of bone
  — evidence of fracture
  — evidence of periosteal reaction
  — trace the length of femur for abnormality
  — check the pelvis
  — look at the soft tissue shadows.

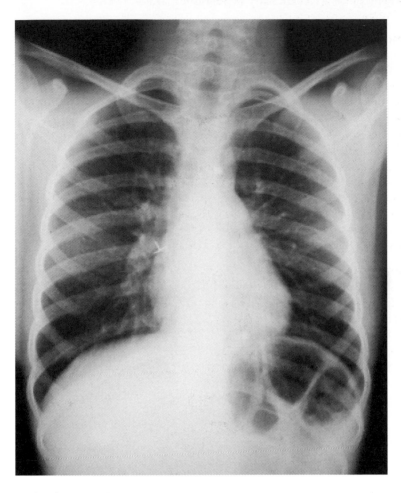

What is the diagnosis?

ANSWER 92

Drawing pin as a foreign body in the right main bronchus.

Comments

- The diagnosis is easy but not all foreign bodies are radio-opaque.
- Always consider the diagnosis in the presence of unilateral wheezing.
- The history may not necessarily be supported by abnormal physical findings, although an intermittent cough is likely.
- Radiologically, the appearance may be unilateral hyperinflation on the affected side, particularly demonstrated on an expiratory film. Total collapse of a segment or lobe is always possible. In both circumstances, the only abnormal physical sign may be tracheal deviation.
- This required removal by rigid bronchoscopy.
- A tracheal foreign body is likely to cause bidirectional stridor.

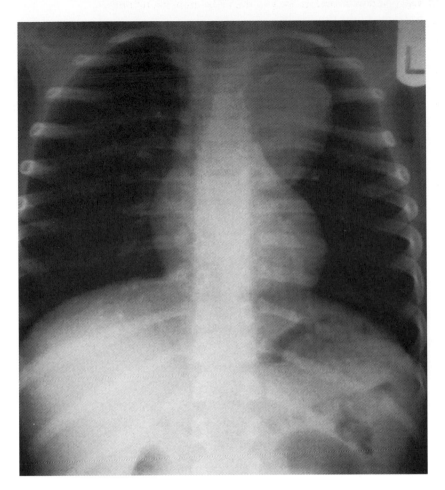

This X-ray was arranged due to a history of nocturnal chest pain.

a) List three abnormal radiological signs.
b) What is the most likely diagnosis?

ANSWER 93

a) Tracheal deviation.
   Splaying of the upper ribs.
   Left posterior mediastinal mass.
   Probable thinning of the upper left ribs.
b) Left thoracic neuroblastoma.

Comments

- This is the classic presentation of a thoracic neuroblastoma arising from the paravertebral chain. The abnormal radiological and clinical features were due to a pressure effect of the tumour.
- The prognosis for total cure is excellent.
- Metastasis at presentation is rare.
- Mediastinal masses have been discussed previously.

Examination tips

- Rehearse the potential presentation of neuroblastoma and the possible investigation results which may be presented, e.g. urinary catecholamines. Like leukaemia, this solid tumour is a frequent visitor to the examination.
- Remember opsoclonus-myoclonus eye movements.

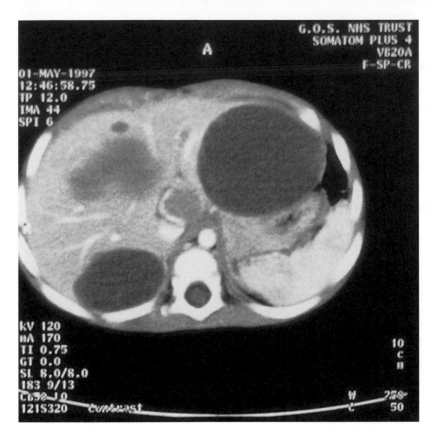

This CT scan was performed as part of a programme of investigations in a toddler with hepatomegaly.

a) What abnormality is noted?
b) List three potential differential diagnoses.
c) Give three corresponding useful investigations to identify the cause.

ANSWER 94

a) Multiple low-density areas throughout the liver ('cyst-like lesions' would also be acceptable).

b) Abscesses (pyogenic or amoebic).
   Tumours (multifocal primary or metastatic).
   Hydatid disease.
   Intrahepatic choledochal cysts.
   Polycystic disease.
   Angiomatous malformations.

c) Biopsy, including culture.
   Hydatid serology.
   Blood and stool cultures.
   Renal ultrasound.
   Liver isotope excretion scan.
   Endoscopic retrograde cholangiopancreatography (ERCP).
   MRI angiogram.

Comments

- In some questions, the diagnosis may be uncertain but an understanding of potential differential diagnoses may be sought.
- The above are some of the potential diagnoses. In fact, the diagnosis was malignancy with a primitive neuroectodermal tumour.
- Hydatid disease was the next leading diagnosis.
- Many infections can home into the liver. Cat scratch disease (CSD) due to *Bartonella henselae* causes similar looking lesions on the ultrasound scan in those who are immuno compromised.

Examination tips

- When asked for a differential diagnosis, list your selection based on the most common or the most likely in the clinical circumstances first.
- When asked for a corresponding number of helpful investigations, give the most diagnostic investigation for each of the differential diagnoses.

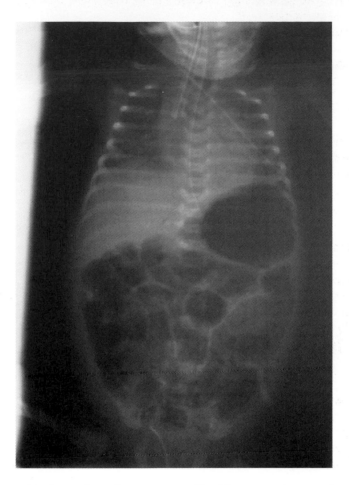

A neonate of 8 days of age became unwell with recurrent apnoeic episodes and abdominal distension. The infant required fluid support. This X-ray was obtained.

a) List all the radiological abnormalities demonstrated.
b) What is the diagnosis?

ANSWER 95

a) Distended loops of bowel.
   Oedematous bowel wall.
   Pneumatosis coli (gas in the bowel wall).
   Portal vein gas.
   Malplaced endotracheal tube.
b) Necrotising enterocolitis.

Comments

- Even though the penetration of the film is not ideal, pneumatosis coli can be definitely identified in the left iliac fossa.
- The presence of portal gas is an ominous sign.
- There is no evidence of visceral perforation yet.
- Always check the position of the endotracheal tube.

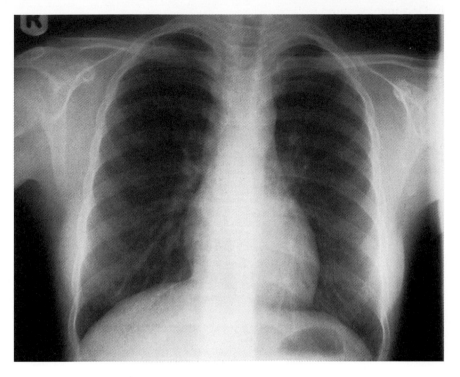

This child was referred to the chest clinic with a Heaf test grade 3. This chest X-ray was performed.

a) What abnormality is demonstrated?
b) What is the relationship to the grade 3 Heaf test?

ANSWER 96

a) Calcified lymph node in the left axilla.
b) Uncertain!

Comments

- Calcification of nodes may occur after chronic infections such as TB and chronic inflammation. Although it is tempting to blame TB, as suggested by the positive Heaf test, there is no other evidence of TB nor any other areas of lymphadenopathy.
- TB nodes around the hilum may be visualised optimally by CT scan.

Examination tips

- Unless the exhortation to look outside the immediate field of interest is followed, it would be easy to miss this presentation. Similar pictures are shown with calcified cervical lymph nodes.

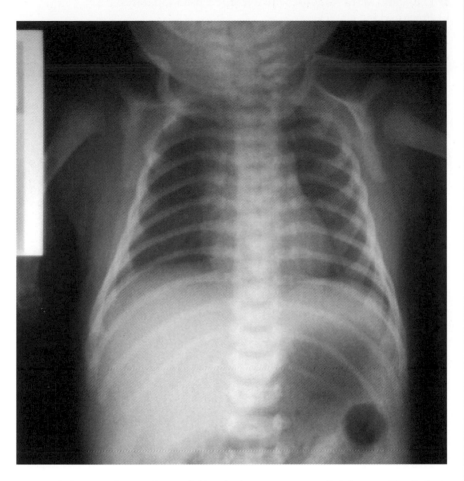

A term baby was born after a difficult non-instrumental delivery. The baby's initial cord gas revealed: pH 7.20, BXs = –15. The baby had a marked caput succadenaeum. Concerns were raised during the first day neonatal examination when a chest X-ray was performed.

a) What clinical feature caused concern?
b) What is the cause?
c) What is the treatment?

ANSWER 97

a) Unilateral Moro response with left-sided pseudoparalysis.
b) Fractured left clavicle.
c) None required – analgesia rarely required.

Comments

- A fracture may occur as part of birth trauma. It is important to feel the clavicle during clinical assessment.
- The fracture must be documented so that incidental finding of evidence of callus formation does not cause concern about child abuse later.
- The differential diagnosis includes brachial plexus nerve injury.

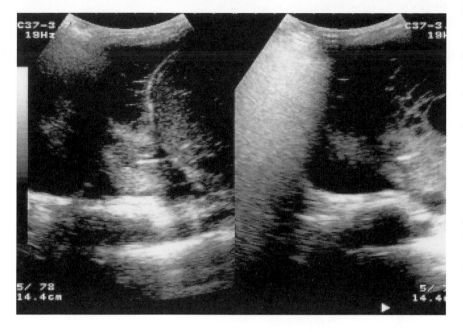

This is an ultrasound of the chest of a boy with a pneumonia which fails to resolve.

What is demonstrated?

ANSWER 98

Fine fibrin collections starting to cause loculation of the pleural fluid during conversion into an empyema.

Comments

Please see diagrammatic representation for orientation:

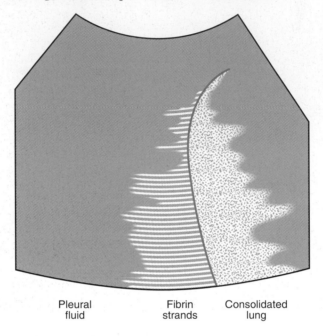

| Pleural fluid | Fibrin strands | Consolidated lung |

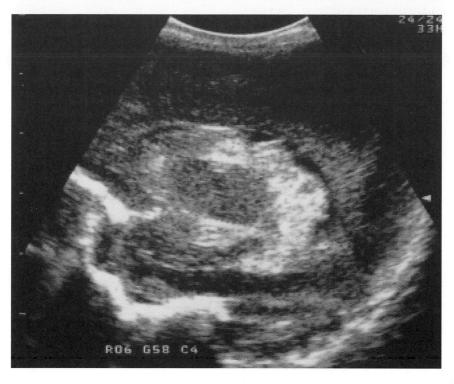

This is a 25-week gestation infant born in poor condition with severe respiratory failure, a coagulopathy, thrombocytopenia and evidence of Group b beta-haemolytic streptococcal septicaemia.

a) What view is shown?
b) What is the diagnosis?

ANSWER 99

a) Parasagittal view of a cranial ultrasound scan.
b) Large intraventricular haemorrhage filling the majority of the lateral ventricle.

Comments

- This demonstrates the bright fresh haemorrhagic echo seen on the scan.
- The clot fills most of the ventricle. It would appear that the ventricle may be starting to dilate, which often occurs after 10–14 days post-haemorrhage.
- There is no definite extraventricular extension.

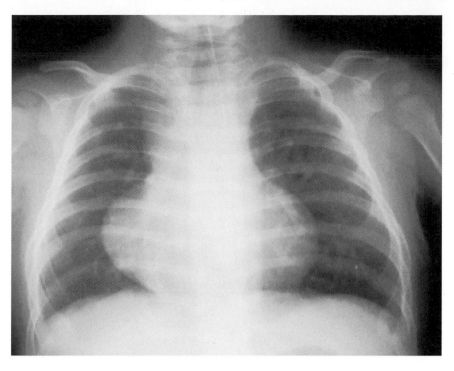

This infant was noted to be cyanosed approximately 4 hours after delivery. No murmurs were audible and the infant was not dysmorphic. The ECG showed right axis deviation, right atrial hypertrophy and right ventricular hypertrophy.

What is the most likely diagnosis?

ANSWER 100

Pulmonary atresia with a ventricular septal defect.

Comments
- This resembles tetralogy of Fallot in some respects, although presentation tends to be earlier.
- There is relative pulmonary oligaemia and the left cardiac border tends to appear longer than that seen with tetralogy of Fallot.
- These children do not squat and do not have profound cyanotic episodes.
- The quoted percentage is 1% of congenital cardiac problems.

Index

Abdominal X-ray
  abdominal neuroblastoma 1, 2
  constipation 125, 126
  Hirschsprung's disease 23, 24
  iatrogenic added shadows 157, 158
  jejunal atresia 9, 10
  necrotising enterocolitis 17, 18, 61, 62, 189, 190
  renal calculus 179, 180
Aicardi syndrome 6
Appendix abscess 151, 152
Arachnoid cyst 44, 169, 170
Aspergilloma 30
Asthma, chronic 109, 110

Back pain 106
Bronchiectasis 91, 92
Bronchiolitis, acute 55, 56
Bronchopneumonia 159, 160
Buckle stress fracture 113, 114

Carbon monoxide poisoning 150
Cerebral atrophy 173, 174
CHARGE syndrome 10, 34
Chest X-ray
  acute bronchiolitis 55, 56
  artefactual radiolucent shadow 69, 70
  bronchopneumonia 159, 160
  chronic asthma 109, 110
  clavicle fracture 193, 194
  cystic fibrosis 35, 36
  cystic lung lesion 29, 30
  empyema 165, 166
  endotracheal tube misplacement 11, 12
  foreign body 171, 172, 183, 184
  hiatus hernia 123, 124
  left ventricular hypertrophy 155, 156
  lobar consolidation/collapse 153, 154
  long line site abnormality 147, 148
  lymph node calcification 191, 192
  lymphocytic interstitial pneumonitis
    (LIP) 81, 82
  mediastinal widening 59, 60
  pleural collections 11, 12, 165, 166
  pneumomediastinum 95, 96
  pulmonary atresia 199, 200
  smoke inhalation pneumonitis 149, 150
  tension pneumothorax 85, 86
  thoracic neuroblastoma 185, 186
  transposition of great arteries 131, 132
  tuberculosis 133, 134
Choanal atresia 33, 34
Choroid plexus tumour 50, 51
Chylothorax 14
Ciliary dyskinesia 92
Clavicle fracture 193, 194
Communicating hydrocephalus 177, 178
Computed tomography
  bronchiectasis 91, 92
  congenital lung cyst 175, 176
  corpus callosum dysgenesis 5, 6
  cystic adenomatoid malformation 89, 90
  empyema 73, 74
  encephalopathy with calcification 167, 168

extradural haematoma 77, 78
  frontal lobe pathology 121, 122, 169, 170
  fronto-parietal cerebral infarct 71, 72
  liver cyst-like lesions 187, 188
  maxillary sinusitis 49, 50
  posterior fossa tumour 31, 32
  retinoblastoma 129, 130
  subarachnoid haemorrhage 141, 142
  thalamic haemorrhage 117, 118
  vein of Galen aneurysmal malformation
    19, 20
  Wilms' tumour 83, 84
Constipation 125, 126
Corpus callosum dysgenesis 5, 6
Cystic adenomatoid malformation 89, 90
Cystic fibrosis 35, 36, 91, 92
Cytomegalovirus infection, congenital 107,
  108

DMSA radioisotope scan 65, 66
'Double bubble' 37, 38
Down's syndrome 38
DTPA radioisotope scan 103, 104
Duodenal atresia 37, 38

Empyema 14, 73, 74, 165, 166, 195, 196
Encephalopathy with calcification 167, 168
Endotracheal tube 157, 158
  misplaced 11, 12
Ependymoma 51
Epiglottitis 40
Extradural haematoma 77, 78

Femur fracture 163, 164
Fetal surgery 172
Foreign body 171, 172, 183, 184
Frontal lobe
  abscess 121, 122
  focal atrophy 169, 170
Frontal sinusitis 15, 16

Growth arrest 113, 114

Haemothorax 14
Hiatus hernia 123, 124
Hip X-ray 101, 102, 181, 182
Hirschsprung's disease 23, 24
HIV infection 82
Hydrocephalus 177, 178

Intracranial tumour
  posterior fossa 31, 32
  supratentorial 50, 51
Intravenous urogram (IVU) 7, 8, 27, 28, 79,
  80
Intraventricular haemorrhage 75, 76, 197,
  198
Intussusception, acute 45, 46

Jejunal atresia 9, 10

Lateral ventricle dilatation 137, 138
Lead poisoning 21, 22
Leptomeningeal cyst 42

Limb X-ray
  femur fracture 163, 164
  growth arrest 113, 114
  lead lines 21, 22
Lissencephaly (pachygyria) 99, 100
Liver cyst-like lesions 188
Liver tumour 187, 188
Lobar consolidation/collapse 153, 154
Long line site abnormality 147, 148
Lung abscess 30
Lung cyst 29, 30, 175, 176
Lymph node calcification 191, 192
Lymphocytic interstitial pneumonitis (LIP) 81, 82

Magnetic resonance imaging (MRI)
  cerebral atrophy 173, 174
  communicating hydrocephalus 177, 178
  hippocampal disease 67, 68
  pachygyria (lissencephaly) 99, 100
  polymicrogyria 57, 58
  spinal haemangioma 105, 106
  sudural haemorrhage 3, 4, 111, 112
Maxillary sinusitis 145, 146
Meatal stenosis 7, 8
Mediastinal widening 59, 60
Medulloblastoma 32
Megaureter 27, 28
Micturating cystourethrogram (MCUG) 8, 97, 98
Mycoplasma pneumoniae infection 159, 160

Necrotising enterocolitis 17, 18, 61, 62, 189, 190
Neonatal cranial ultrasound
  congenital cytomegalovirus infection 107, 108
  intracranial cyst-like lesion 43, 44
  intraventricular haemorrhage 75, 76, 197, 198
  lateral ventricle dilatation 137, 138
  periventricular leucomalacia 53, 54
  prominent third ventricle 119, 120
Neonate
  clavicle fracture 193, 194
  cystic adenomatous malformation 89, 90
  duodenal atresia 37, 38
  encephalopathy with calcification 167, 168
  frontoparietal cerebral infarct 71, 72
  jejunal atresia 9, 10
  long line site abnormality 147, 148
  necrotising enterocolitis 17, 18, 189, 190
  pachygyria (lissencephaly) 99, 100
  pleural collection 11, 12
  pulmonary atresia 199, 200
  sudural haemorrhage 111, 112
  superior pneumomediastinum 95, 96
  thalamic necrosis 117, 118
  transposition of great arteries 131, 132
  vein of Galen malformation 19, 20, 43, 44
  see also Neonatal cranial ultrasound
Neuroblastoma
  abdominal 1, 2
  thoracic 185, 186

Neurofibromatosis type 1 51
Non-accidental injury 25, 26, 128, 164

Obstructive uropathy 7, 8
Osteopenic bones 113, 114

Pachygyria (lissencephaly) 99, 100
Partial epilepsy 67, 68
Percutaneous long line site abnormality 147, 148
Periventricular leucomalacia 53, 54
Perthes' disease 101, 102
Pleural collection 11, 12
Pleural effusion 165, 166
Pneumococcal meningitis 49, 50
Pneumomediastinum 95, 96
Pneumonia 154, 195, 196
Polymicrogyria 57, 58
Porencephalic cyst 44
Posterior fossa tumour 31, 32
Posterior urethral valves 162
Preterm infant
  iatrogenic added shadows on abdominal X-ray 157, 158
  intraventricular haemorrhage 197, 198
  lateral ventricle dilatation 137, 138
  misplaced endotracheal tube 11, 12
  necrotising enterocolitis 61, 62
  respiratory disease 143, 144
  tension pneumothorax 85, 86
  umbilical arterial line aberrant positioning 93, 94
Pulmonary atresia 199, 200
Pyothorax 14

Radioisotope scan
  renal scarring 65, 66
  vesicoureteric reflux 103, 104
Renal calculus 179, 180
Renal cysts 80
Renal scarring 65, 66
Respiratory distress syndrome (surfactant deficient hyaline membrane disease) 144
Retinoblastoma 129, 130
Retro-orbital abscess 115, 116
Retropharyngeal oedema/abscess 39, 40

Sickle cell disease 155, 156
Sinusitis 15, 16, 49, 50, 145, 146
Skull fracture 25, 26, 41, 42, 127, 128
Skull X-ray
  linear fracture 25, 26
  sinusitis 15, 16, 145, 146
  wormian bones 135, 136
Slipped upper femoral epiphysis 102, 181, 182
Small bowel obstruction 87, 88
Smoke inhalation pneumonitis 149, 150
Spinal haemangioma 105, 106
Streptococcal sepsis 144
Subarachnoid haemorrhage 141, 142
Subdural haemorrhage 3, 4, 111, 112, 142

Subglottic narrowing 139, 140
Surfactant deficient hyaline membrane
    disease (respiratory distress
    syndrome) 144

Tension pneumothorax 85, 86
Thalamic necrosis 117, 118
Third ventricle pathology 119, 120
Thymoma 59, 60
Tracheo-oesophageal fistula 53, 54
Transposition of great arteries 131, 132
Tuberculosis 30, 82, 133, 134, 192
Tuberose sclerosis 51

Ultrasound
    empyema 195, 196
    see also Neonatal cranial ultrasound

Umbilical arterial line 157, 158
    aberrant positioning 93, 94
Umbilical venous line 157, 158

Vein of Galen malformation 19, 20, 43, 44
Ventricular index 138
Ventricular septal defect
    with pulmonary atresia 199, 200
    with transposition of great arteries 131,
    132
Vesicoureteric reflux 97, 98, 103, 104, 161,
    162

Wilms' tumour 83, 84
Wormian bones 135, 136

X-linked hypophosphataemic rickets 47, 48

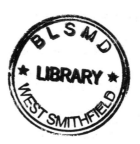